Customer-Driven Healthcare: QFD for Process Improvement and Cost Reduction

Also available from ASQ Quality Press

How to Use Patient Satisfaction Data to Improve Health Care Quality
Ralph Bell, Ph.D. and Michael J. Krivich, M.H.A., C.H.E.

How to Use Control Charts in HealthCare
D. Lynn Kelley

The Handbook for Managing Change in Health Care
ASQ Health Care Series, Chip Caldwell, editor

Mentoring Strategic Change in Health Care: An Action Guide
Chip Caldwell

Healthcare Performance Measurement: Systems Design and Evaluation
Vahé A. Kazandjian and Terry R. Lied

Root Cause Analysis: Simplified Tools and Techniques
Bjørn Andersen

Quality Function Deployment: A Practitioner's Approach
James L. Bossert

Quality Function Deployment: Linking a Company with its Customers
Ronald G. Day

Measuring Customer Satisfaction: Survey Design, Use, and Statistical Analysis Methods Bob E. Hayes

Customer Satisfaction Measurement and Management
Earl Naumann and Kathleen Giel

Statistical Quality Control Using EXCEL (with software)
Steven M. Zimmerman and Marjorie L. Icenogle

To request a complimentary catalog of ASQ Quality Press publications, call 800-248-1946, or visit our website at qualitypress.asq.org .

Customer-Driven Healthcare: QFD for Process Improvement and Cost Reduction

by
Ed Chaplin, M.D.
John Terninko, Ph.D.

ASQ Quality Press
Milwaukee, Wisconsin

Library of Congress Cataloging-in-Publication Data

Chaplin, Ed, 1945–
    Customer driven healthcare: QFD for process improvement and cost reduction/Ed
Chaplin, John Terninko.
        p. cm.
    Includes bibliographical references and index.
    ISBN 0-87389-471-5 (alk. paper)
        1. Medical care—United States—Quality control. 2. Quality function deployment. 3. Medical care—United States—
Cost effectiveness. 4. Medical care—United States—Cost control. I. Terninko, John. II. Title.

RA394 .C47 2000
362.1'068'5—dc21   99-056126

10 9 8 7 6 5 4 3 2 1

ISBN 0-87389-471-5

Acquisitions Editor: Ken Zielske
Project Editor: Annemieke Koudstaal
Production Administrator: Shawn Dohogne
Special Marketing Representative: David Luth

ASQ Mission: The American Society for Quality advances individual and organizational performance excellence worldwide by providing opportunities for learning, quality improvement, and knowledge exchange.

Attention: Bookstores, Wholesalers, Schools and Corporations:
ASQ Quality Press books, videotapes, audiotapes, and software are available at quantity discounts with bulk purchases for business, educational, or instructional use. For information, please contact ASQ Quality Press at 800-248-1946, or write to ASQ Quality Press, P.O. Box 3005, Milwaukee, WI 53201-3005.

To place orders or to request a free copy of the ASQ Quality Press Publications Catalog, including ASQ membership information, call 800-248-1946. Visit our web site at www.asq.org. or qualitypress.asq.org.

Printed in the United States of America

 Printed on acid-free paper

American Society for Quality

ASQ

Quality Press
611 East Wisconsin Avenue
Milwaukee, Wisconsin 53202
Call toll free 800-248-1946
www.asq.org
qualitypress.asq.org
standardsgroup.asq.org

To our parents,
To our teachers, whom we "regard in this art
as equal to our parents,"[1] and

To Peggy and Candy, companions, wives,
a sister and a sister-in-law.

We thank James Bruer and Joe Miller
for contributions to the appendixes.

---

1. From the oath of Hippocrates.

Table of Contents

List of Illustrations

Part I

Healthcare Perspective

Chapter 1

The Context
and the Challenge

Upon completion of this chapter, you will have:

- An overview of quality function deployment (QFD)

- A sense of where QFD fits into the total quality management (TQM) spectrum

- An overview of the text

*E*fficient and effective patient-focused systems to generate quality outcomes and patient satisfaction . . .*" This phrase or some variation is repeated so often today, it has become a healthcare mantra. Experience, however, indicates that the principle is more easily articulated than accomplished.

How many healthcare organizations really listen to their customers without filtering what the customer says through a screen of the organization's own internal concerns and needs? How many healthcare organizations that do listen to their customers are able to respond in a way that effectively improves the performance of everyday tasks and processes? The future will belong to healthcare organizations that can continuously reinvent processes that adapt to today's rapidly changing environment.

Compare the relative inefficiency of our ability to diagnose, treat, and innovate within the systems that deliver healthcare to our increasingly effective ability to diagnose and treat acute medical problems and to the phenomenal innovations that are occurring in biotechnology. If there was a way to generate similarly effective processes for the diagnosis, management, and innovation of healthcare delivery, you would probably want to know about it. In this text, you will be introduced to a collection of processes that form an integrated system to accomplish this goal.

The services in acute medicine and biotechnology emanate from the same fundamental organizational theory—the unified theory of the *cell* as a system. This book presents a brief overview of the cell as a model for a successful organization, and then describes *quality function deployment (QFD)* as a set of practices and tools used to design services that, like the cell, are self-organizing and self-regulating.

In the healthcare industry, we tend to see ourselves as being on the cutting edge when it comes to applying scientific discoveries to the technical aspects of delivering medical care. However, we are relatively slow to adopt tools that improve the quality of service. The tools of *total quality management (TQM),* which evolved in Japan, were first introduced to the United States through the manufacturing industries during the 1980s. Many service industries adopted the theories of TQM to their needs before the healthcare industry had even become aware of TQM's benefits. Similarly, QFD (a more recently developed quality management strategy) first appeared in this country in the automobile industries and has since been adapted for the service industries. The application of QFD provides a standard set of practices that, when used, improve satisfaction with healthcare delivery.

WHAT IS QFD AND WHERE DOES IT FIT?

QFD is a set of tools linked as steps to form a process. The tools of QFD define targets, describe measurable feedback by which to navigate toward these targets, and describe key actions necessary to reach these targets. QFD, by design,

- Goes outside organization boundaries to capture and rank information from customers and the environment

- Translates this information into organizational targets and measures

- Organizes the activity of people around these targets and identifies feedback measures to produce specific services that generate value for the customer

A case example is presented in detail to show how QFD was used to redesign a service within a rehabilitation hospital. At a very high schematic level, rehabilitation services begin with an *initial assessment* that identifies the patient/customer's current physical capacity, his or her desired targets or goals, physical and social barriers to achieving these targets, and the assets available for overcoming these barriers (Figure 1.1). A series of *actions* or therapies are carried out. Cognitive and physical capacities are reassessed, and these *reassessments* are used to modify treatment plans and to guide discharge planning.

Like most hospitals accredited by the Joint Commission on Accreditation of Healthcare Organizations, the hospital in our study used patient-satisfaction surveys, the basic quality tools (Nayatani et al. 1988), and specialized outcome assessment tools such as the functional independence measure (FIM) (Granger et al. 1990) for quality assurance and continuous quality improvement (CQI) activities (Figure 1.2). These are tools used to measure results. QFD, in contrast, is a process to plan and design the delivery of services. QFD makes extensive use of the new quality tools—particularly affinity grouping, tree diagrams, and matrices—to identify qualities demanded by customers, to identify characteristics and performance measures of these qualities, and to link these performance measures to the key organizational functions and critical tasks that are necessary to satisfy the demanded qualities.

Quality assurance, CQI, quality planning, and QFD are all encompassed under the larger umbrella known as TQM (Figure 1.2). The figure is not meant to imply that quality planning, quality assurance, CQI, and QFD constitute all of TQM. Nor does the figure imply that QFD and CQI are mutually exclusive. For example, outcomes from CQI monitors can be used to further modify design and performance measures identified with QFD, which can then become CQI indicators.

Most evidence and examples of QFD's effectiveness as a design process are for products rather than services. Many applications for medical products have been com-

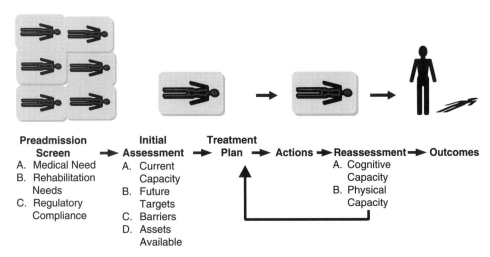

Preadmission
Screen ➔ Initial Assessment ➔ Treatment Plan ➔ Actions ➔ Reassessment ➔ Outcomes

A. Medical Need
B. Rehabilitation Needs
C. Regulatory Compliance

A. Current Capacity
B. Future Targets
C. Barriers
D. Assets Available

A. Cognitive Capacity
B. Physical Capacity

Figure 1.1. Inpatient rehabilitation service as a process. The service line can be seen as a series of assessments, actions (treatments), followed by reassessments and adjustment of actions to produce desired outcomes.

Source: Journal on Quality Improvement (Oakbrook, Ill.: Joint Commission on Accreditation of Healthcare Organizations, 1999), 300–315. Reprinted with permission.

pleted in areas such as dental hardware and compounds, surgical instruments, casts, tapes, and orthopedic hardware. These medical-hardware applications of QFD can be analyzed and understood by reading books on QFD for products (Terninko 1995). However, the limited number of service examples found in the public domain, word-of-mouth stories, and personal experiences indicates that the principles learned from QFD product applications are important in service industries as well, including the service area of healthcare. For example, QFD was used by a Japanese translation company, resulting in the development of a process flow that reduced turnaround time. "Japan Business Consultants has continued to grow in both revenues and the number of quality materials it handles" (Mazur 1996). Since 1988, North American software organizations have been applying QFD for software development (Zultner 1992). Leading firms, such as AT&T Bell Laboratories, Hewlett-Packard, and IBM, have reported improved software products and improved software deployment through the use of task deployment. Task deployment is very important in healthcare applications. Through the use of QFD, Rehab Concepts, a physical rehabilitation facility, identified a significant missing customer segment. As a result, the facility became the leading provider of physical rehabilitation for industrial accidents in the state of Massachusetts (case in Appendix G). New England Memorial Hospital used QFD for the design of their new emergency room. Two breakthrough concepts resulted: one was to provide the space necessary for protected transfer of patients from an ambulance, and the other was to provide a convenient path for patients leaving the hospital via an ambulance (case in Appendix F).

A fundamental difference between the traditional manufacturing design process and the design process using QFD is the allocation of time, money, and staff. Traditionally, the allocation of resources begins modestly and increases to a peak as problems and

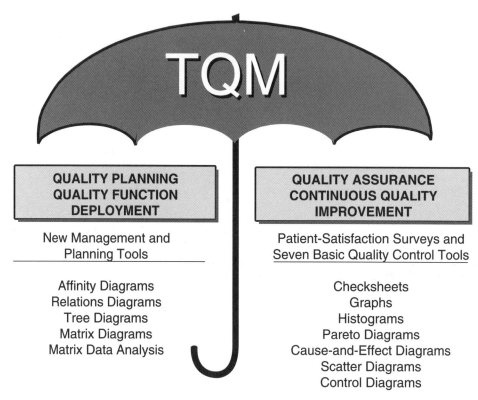

Figure 1.2. Total quality management activities. Quality planning, quality assurance, continuous quality improvement, and quality function deployment (QFD) are represented as part of a larger set of tools and strategies under the total quality management (TQM) umbrella. Quality assurance and continuous quality improvement activities focus on results. The tools include checksheets, graphs, histograms, Pareto diagrams, cause-and-effect diagrams, scatter diagrams, and control charts and diagrams. In contrast, quality planning and quality function deployment focus on design. They utilize new management and planning tools including affinity diagrams, relation diagrams, tree diagrams, matrix diagrams, and matrix data analysis.

Source: Journal on Quality Improvement (Oakbrook, Ill.: Joint Commission on Accreditation of Health-care Organizations, 1999), 300–315. Reprinted with permission.

breakdowns requiring corrective action occur (after production or deployment of the service) (Figure 1.3). In contrast, QFD embodies the philosophy of "doing it right the first time" by allocating more time and resources up front.

Several years ago, Ford Motor Company tracked the allocation of resources as the number of engineering changes per unit. A plot of the number of engineering changes per unit of time for a traditional design project showed a peak of activity just before the product goes to market (Figure 1.4). This was the result of building a prototype to identify failure modes. The process was repeated several times. During the 1980s, each new concept for a car required an average of 3.7 engineering changes. Once production

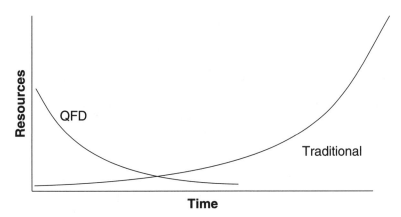

Figure 1.3. Allocation of resources. In traditional design and implementation projects, the allocation of resources increases as a function of time right up to implimentation. In QFD, in contrast, there is an allocation of more resources up front and less are needed at the time of producing a product or delivering a service.

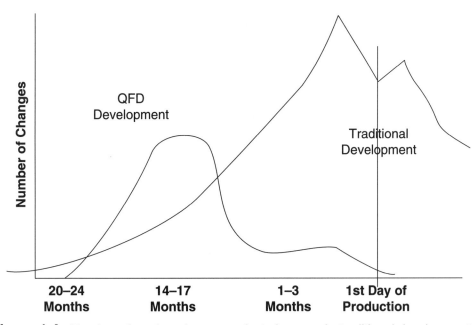

Figure 1.4. Number of engineering or product changes. In traditional development, the number of engineering changes per unit of time increases just prior to production and continues for a period after production as customers identify defects. In QFD, in contrast, the peak of engineering changes occurs 14 to 17 months prior to the first day of production.

Source: Adapted from L. P. Sullivan, "Quality Function Deployment," *Quality Progress* (June 1996). Reprinted with permission.

started, there was an initial decline in the number of engineering changes, but this proved only temporary as customers discovered errors in function. When QFD was used as a basis for the design process, the curve for the number of changes managed over a period of time peaked 14 to 17 months prior to the start of production. This first peak represented resources expended in solving the major aspects in the design process and dealing with conflicts that were likely to arise early in the design phase. Because most changes were made prior to the start of production, the net result was a significant saving of resources.

Although we know of no comparable data for service industries, consider how much of your day-to-day management activities are spent tracking "defects" in service processes and then instituting "corrective actions." Surveys have suggested that health-care managers expend 40 percent of their time engaged in addressing service commitment breakdowns and conflict resolution. (Lippitt 1982).

QFD: A HIGH-LEVEL VIEW

The QFD process begins by identifying the customer. The process then identifies customer concerns and requirements. This information is used to define measures for these requirements, and these measures are used to design processes and to implement changes in day-to-day operations that satisfy these requirements (Figure 1.5).

The variation of QFD that will be presented here is illustrated by Figure 1.6. This process follows a previously described, six-step format for QFD (Terninko 1995; Mazur 1996):

Step 1	Capturing the voice of the customer
Step 2	Quality deployment
Step 3	Function deployment
Step 4	Failure mode deployment
Step 5	New process deployment
Step 6	Task deployment

The QFD team identifies and translates customer requirements into organizational functions and tasks that will generate customer assessments of satisfaction. The output

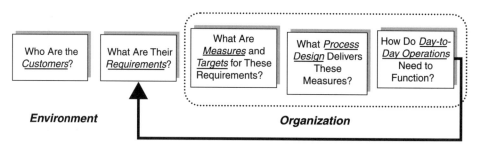

Figure 1.5. QFD as a process. QFD begins by identifying who the customers are and then what these customers' requirements are. Next, measures of these requirements and targets from these measures are identified. These measures are then used to design processes to deliver customer requirements and to achieve targeted measures by identifying key functions and tasks and changing operations.

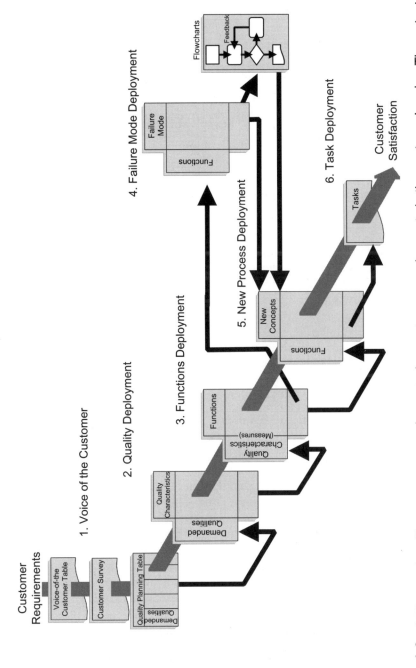

Figure 1.6. QFD overview. The process starts by capturing customer requirements in the customer's voice. The output of each step becomes the input to a table or matrix tool for the next step of the process. This linkage ensures that qualities perceived as important by customers are translated and remain coupled to organizational performance measures, key functions, and critical tasks as the organization designs or redesigns systems to deliver demanded qualities.

Source: Journal on Quality Improvement (Oakbrook, Ill.: Joint Commission on Accreditation of Healthcare Organizations, 1999), 300–315. Reprinted with permission.

of each step in the process becomes the input to a matrix tool or table for the next step. The next several paragraphs present a brief overview of QFD as a process.

Step 1: Capturing the Voice of the Customer

Fifteen to twenty customers are interviewed in the field. Data captured in these interviews is placed into a *voice-of-the-customer table (VOCT)* to identify customer needs. A *demanded quality* is identified by asking *why* the customer uses the services.

Demanded qualities are then used to design a *survey* that is mailed to a larger group of customers. Data captured by interviewing customers is *qualitative* in nature. The survey provides the opportunity to obtain *quantitative* data about customer wants, rankings for these wants, and feedback of how the organization is perceived in satisfying these wants relative to its competitors.

The results of the survey are then entered into a *quality-planning table.* This table lists demanded qualities, the importance ratings of these demanded qualities from the customer's perspective, and the customer's competitive ranking of the organization's services compared to other providers. In addition, the quality-planning table will be used to set targets for improvement and to choose which demanded qualities will be carried to the next step.

> *Step 1 identifies the customer's wants and needs, as well as the organization's targets for improving its service to meet these needs.*

Step 2: Quality Deployment

The demanded qualities that are identified as important from the customer's perspective and that provide the greatest opportunity for improvement in the organization's services become a target for that service and are entered into the *demanded quality/performance matrix* (Figure 1.6). Demanded qualities, which are in the language of the customer, are translated into performance measures that the healthcare organization can use to evaluate alternative systems and procedures for satisfying the customer's needs.

> *Step 2 identifies the quantitative performance measures that will be used to evaluate whether or not demanded qualities are delivered.*

Step 3: Function Deployment

The more important performance measures identified in Step 2 become the input to the *performance measures/functions matrix* (Figure 1.6). This matrix translates performance measures into the functions necessary to satisfy the customer. Every organization is designed to perform some primary function and necessary secondary functions. The importance of the performance measures is remapped to these functions.

The Joint Commission on the Accreditation of Healthcare Organizations is moving beyond checking the adequacy of facilities, beyond checking policies and procedures, and beyond certifying that quality assurance processes are in place. The introduction of the ORYX™ initiative will integrate sets of continuous performance measures into the accreditation process (www.jcaho.com). We will be presenting a comprehensive case example of QFD. However, if a set of performance measures was already defined, it could be the input to Step 3.

> *Step 3 identifies the key functions that the organization needs to perform to generate the desired quality for the systems and procedures necessary to satisfy customer needs.*

Step 4: Failure Mode Deployment

The key functions identified in Step 3 become input to the rows of a *function/failure mode matrix* (Figure 1.6). This matrix is used to identify key failure modes for the functions. The weak points provide an opportunity to incorporate innovative change and feedback measures to enhance the reliability and robustness of the service.

Step 4 identifies the key failure modes that may be experienced by the functions.

There are other tools that can be used to identify potential sources of failure, including *tables*—such as *solutions tables* and *failure-mode-and-effects-analysis (FMEA) tables* (Figure 1.7)—and *trees*—such as *fault tree diagrams* and *management-oversight-and-risk-tree (MORT) analysis* (Figure 1.8). Along with the functions/failure mode matrix, these tools will be used with increasing frequency by healthcare organizations in the near future. They are tools for root cause analysis required by the Joint Commission on the Accreditation of Healthcare Organizations and for their sentinel event initiative. In the QFD process, these tools are used to identify potential modes of failure while designing a process or to search for the root cause of possible breakdowns when redesigning a system after deployment.

Traditionally, root cause or sentinel event analysis begins with a clear statement and identification of a failure that has already occurred. During the solution phase of root cause analysis, the essential features of potential solutions are defined. A robust root cause process involves the identification of key qualities for a solution, quantitative measures of these qualities, and deployment of the solution. As you will see, root cause analysis correlates closely with Step 4 of the QFD process. When applying QFD to design systems, these tools are used to identify failure modes before the failure occurs. Each of the failure analysis tools is discussed in more detail in Part 2 of this text.

Step 5: New Process Deployment

The highest-ranking functions from Step 3 become input for the rows of a *function/new concepts matrix*. New concepts for performing these functions and concepts for overcoming weak points identified in Step 4 become the starting point. Concepts are drawn on a process flowchart, and key tasks are identified. The outputs of this matrix are new concepts for processes and a ranking of all the alternatives.

Step 5 chooses the best overall design for the key functions necessary to deliver services the customer needs.

Step 6: Task Deployment

The selected concepts are broken down into necessary tasks. Tasks that are critical to the key functions are identified from the process flowchart from the preceding selected concept. Critical tasks are placed into a task-deployment table.

Step 6 identifies who will do what, when, where, why, and how, as well as measures and costs of the tasks critical to the delivery of qualities demanded by the customer.

Each of the preceding steps is more fully described later in the text, first as part of an actual case example and then as a step-by-step process to guide a team through the QFD process. The book is organized into two parts, with the second part following the step-by-step, workbook format.

Solutions Table

Problem	Cause	Proposed Solution	Actions
Call Light Not Used to Call for Assistance When Needing to Go to the Bathroom	Patient Confused Urinary Incontinence and Urgency	Frequent Toileting of Confused Patients and Patients with Urinary Frequency	Staff Education and Feedback Measures for Effectiveness
Side Rails Not Up	Patient Not Assessed as Fall Risk Policies and Procedures Not Followed by Staff		

Figure 1.7. Root-cause-analysis tools: tables. The solutions and failure-mode-and-effects-analysis tables are two strategies that use tables as tools for identifying the root causes for breakdowns in organizational products or services.

Failure-Mode-and-Effects-Analysiss

ITEM Function	Potential Failure Mode	Potential Effects of Failures	SEV	Potential Causes of Failure	OCC	Current Design Controls	DET	RPN	Recommended Actions	Responsibility Target for Completion
Preadmission Assessment	Confustion on Part of Team	Less Available Resources	2	Inaccurate Data / Missing Data / Miscommunication / Unnecessary Data	5 / 4 / 4 / 4	Informal "Gotcha" "Victim" Marketing Meeting	4	40		
		Wrong Treatment	4	Inaccurate Data / Missing Data / Miscommunication / Unnecessary Data	5 / 4 / 4 / 4	Occurrence Reports / Quality Concerns / Chart Audits / CM Survey	4	80		
		Missed Treatment (Unidentified Problem)	4	Inaccurate Data / Missing Data / Miscommunication / Unnecessary Data / Incomplete Tasks	5 / 4 / 4 / 4 / 5	Occurrence Reports / Quality Concerns / Chart Audits / CM Survey	4	80		
		Rework	4	Inaccurate Data / Missing Data / Miscommunication / Faded Expectations	4 / 4 / 4 / 2	Productivity Tracking	4	64		
	Condition Not Monitored	Missed Treatment (Unidentified Problem)	5	Inaccurate Data / Missing Data / Miscommunication / Unnecessary Data	5 / 4 / 4 / 4	Occurrence Reports / Quality Concerns / Chart Audits / CM Survey	4	100	Educate Staff in Use of Quality Concerns and Collect Actual Data	2 Weeks, Clinical Department Managers
		Wrong Treatment	5	Inaccurate Data / Missing Data / Miscommunication / Unnecessary Data	5 / 4 / 4 / 4	Occurrence Reports / Quality Concerns / Chart Audits / CM Survey	4	100	Educate Staff in Use of Quality Concerns and Collect Actual Data	2 Weeks, Clinical Department Managers
Initial Assessment on Admission										

Figure 1.7. *Continued.*

13

Fault Tree Analysis

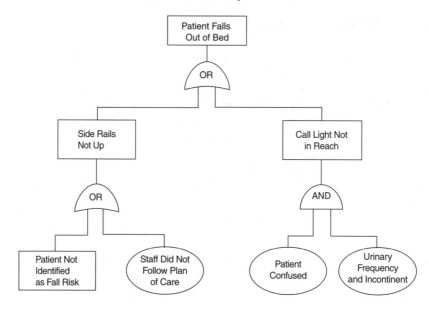

Management-Oversight-and-Risk-Tree Analysis

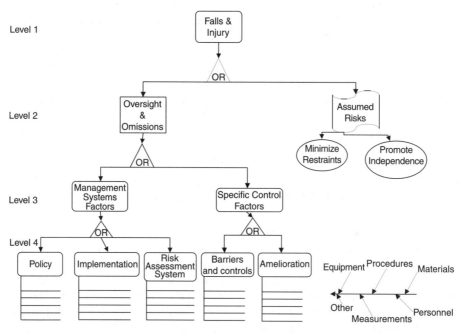

Figure 1.8. Root-cause-analysis tools: trees. Fault tree analysis and management-oversight-and-risk-tree analysis are two root cause strategies that employ trees to identify the source of breakdowns in organizational products or services.

OVERVIEW OF THE TEXT

Part 1: The Healthcare Perspective

Part 1 presents some background, an overview of QFD, and a brief example of a QFD application. *Chapter 1* presents an overview of QFD and of the book.

The design of the book takes into account the process by which we change and learn. We are more open to change and the incorporation of new ideas once we conceptually and experientially encounter the limitations of our current ways. Therefore, *chapter 2* discusses some presuppositions embodied within the culture of healthcare and how they are barriers to actualizing efficient and effective patient-focused systems. The chapter touches on the area of judgment and decision making. This brief section is not meant to solve the controversies between the different schools of thought in this area; rather, it illustrates and emphasizes how our past experience shapes current interpretations and influences choices for action.

We are more effective at grasping and retaining new learning if we can relate the new concepts to familiar structures, relationships, internal maps, and the embodied frameworks we already have. *Chapter 3* presents the living cell as a model of an organization. The biotechnologist's capacity for innovation and the physician's capacity for intelligent and decisive action in acute medical crises are based on this model, components of which are built on distinctions learned in high-school biology and are familiar to all healthcare workers. This model of the cell is used as a framework to introduce important distinctions for the successful implementation of QFD projects. Understanding this framework will enable leaders, managers, and workers in healthcare, particularly people in clinical disciplines, to grasp the distinctions of QFD in a way that promotes insights into key relations and concepts. This chapter is not intended to present a new theory of organizations. Many managers in healthcare are clinicians who, because they were good clinicians, were promoted to managers. Many are without any formal training in management or management systems. The goal of this chapter is to introduce a simple model or schema using terminology already familiar to healthcare workers to build a common background and a context within which to introduce the distinctions important to the QFD process. The management literature is filled with biological metaphors as models for organizations these days, and chapter 3 is consistent with that trend.

For 75 percent to 80 percent of the population, the most effective way of learning is visual: "a picture is worth a thousand words." Pictures allow the viewer to quickly grasp important sets of relations and to understand them as multiple parts of an integrated whole. *Chapter 4* shows us a case study that is a picture of QFD as an integrated system. The case example resulted in a twofold rise in the rate of referrals for the service.

Part 2: Step-by-Step Healthcare QFD

We are at our best in learning and changing behaviors when we are in action. Part 2 of the book is a detailed presentation of the steps used in the chapter 4 case study, but in a workbook format. The workbook is a step-by-step map for a team to practice designing and deploying either a learning example or an actual QFD project. A series of concepts and tools to design or redesign a service is introduced and then practiced. Each step is described in detail. The description includes an example that is followed by an exercise. This provides an opportunity for the design team to actually practice the step. Clean copies of worksheets for key steps are provided in Appendix A. Some historical perspective, experiential strategies, and rationale for the steps in QFD are also provided. The biological model presented earlier is used to identify key concepts and relationships.

The text touches on the four elements of what Demming called profound knowledge:

* Appreciation for systems

* Understanding variation

* A theory of knowledge—how people learn

* A theory of psychology—why people behave as they do

Our goal is to expand awareness and build a capacity for action, not just to present the latest technique. The text also includes several appendixes. These appendixes include blank worksheets, additional details about related strategies referred to in the text, and more case examples. Appendix F reports on a hospital's first experience using the principles of QFD to order priorities. Appendix G describes how this same hospital then used the more formal aspects of QFD to design a service. Appendix H gives brief descriptions of cases in healthcare-related settings where QFDs have been reported to be successful.

To the new initiate, QFD may seem overwhelmingly difficult and complex. So does chess. Like chess, QFD embodies a finite set of rules for action and historical strategies that define and guide a field of possible actions. How these actions unfold and the quality of the results are functions of the skill of the practitioner and the complexity and competitiveness of the environment. Like chess, familiarity with rules, strategies, and successful outcomes improves with practice.

For example, an experienced pulmonologist who is listening to a patient's chest hears not only the noises of breathing, but many different categories of sound—some clear, some coarse, some crackling, some with inspiratory wheezes or expiratory wheezes, and so on. Each sound implies a different status for the respiratory system and calls for different interventions to improve function and restore the health of the patient. As a beginning medical student, the pulmonologist learned a set of abstract concepts and then practiced listening for them. At first, he or she could not differentiate among the sounds. With practice, the student learned to hear the nuances. What were initially abstract terms in a textbook or lecture become distinguishable entities in practice. This enables the pulmonologist to behave in new ways and to further increase his or her powers of observation and intervention. It is hoped that this book will help the reader in much the same way.

The promise to the reader is that if you engage in the exercises and practices presented in this text your capacity to diagnose and treat organizational malaise and inefficiency will be greatly enhanced. This claim can be made in part because of the power of the QFD tools but also because the use of this process will empower you with a new perspective of your organization's structure and function. Using a simple model of the cell to make explicit the essential components necessary for sustaining all living systems, you will be given a clear sense of the three fundamental challenges that every organization faces and how breakdowns in meeting these challenges are the root causes of organizational inefficiencies and failures. You will also have a map of the basic cycle by which human beings coordinate actions and exchange value with others. Together, this model and map provide a lens for focusing your diagnosis of the breakdowns that befall our human social structures and organizations. Finally, you will have the opportunity to practice using a set of tools from QFD that will allow you to "treat" these breakdowns by identifying what is missing, setting new targets, and designing processes that allow more healthy and efficient practices to emerge.

Chapter 2

Barriers to Patient-Focused Services and Systems

Upon completion of this chapter, you will have a sense of:

- Historical barriers to change

- How our past experiences and expectations for the future shape our perception of the present

- How standard processes or algorithms enhance consistency and help us overcome barriers

HISTORICAL BARRIERS TO CHANGE

Healthcare has a number of historical barriers that impede the incorporation of the voice of the customer into the delivery of its services. First, healthcare has evolved within a strong tradition of paternalism—the doctor or nurse knows what is best for the patient. Informed consent as a standard practice is a relatively recent phenomenon. Twenty years ago, patients who might have had a disease such as multiple sclerosis or cancer routinely were not told that these diagnoses were suspected. Providers thought that such knowledge was not good for the patient, as it might adversely influence the patient's behavior.

Healthcare also has an unfortunate and strong tradition of holding the customer responsible for unsuccessful treatment. For example, when treatments or procedures do not work and the healthcare provider becomes frustrated, labels such as "poor protoplasm," "crock," "noncompliant," and so on are sometimes applied. Although denial and noncompliance are major problems in some disorders—such as addiction—these labels have been and still are used directly and covertly in a wide variety of healthcare settings. The net effect is to make the healthcare provider right and the patient/customer wrong.

THE NATURE OF PERCEPTION

Healthcare is steeped in the fundamental premises of Western science. These include:

- *Realism:* the assumption that we see the world as it exists without distortion

- *Separateness:* the belief that local events have local and separate causes

- *Inductive prediction:* the faith that logical conclusions can be predicted from consistent observations

When faced with a problem, we step back and separate ourselves from it. We gather objective data, reduce the problem to its components, construct an accurate and objective representation, and predict what actions will obtain the desired results. This strategy is the strength of the Western scientific tradition. It underlies medical diagnosis and treatment, and, most of the time, it is very effective. By its nature, however, this method inherently slows and self-limits our capacity to change.

Inductive prediction is based on constructing a model of the future that comes from the past. This generates a perception of the future that is dependent on the past. However, one thing seems clear in today's rapidly changing healthcare environment. The future will likely be radically different from the past, and the future will belong to those who can rapidly change and innovate, not to those who blindly cling to the past.

These observations on the limitations of Western science have been made before (Kuhn 1996; Manturana and Varela 1988; Pribram 1991). Still, many of the effects of our presuppositions and cultural conditioning are far more subtle and more difficult to recognize. Consider, for example, the fact that each of us has a blind spot in our field of vision. This blind spot results from a gap in the retinal sensors where the optic nerve pierces the back of the eye. Yet, we do not go around with a hole in our field of vision. Why not?

Our visual system fills in the blind spot. To prove this point, experimenters had subjects stare at a distant screen with one eye open and one eye shut (Ramachandran on 1993). In this way, the blind spot was located and outlined (Figure 2.1a). The experimenters then made a thick, colored ring (Figure 2.1b) of sufficient size to stimulate the receptors around the margins of the blind spot but not the blind spot itself. When the ring was placed over the area of the blind spot, subjects report that they saw not a ring but a colored dot or disk such as in Figure 2.1c. This demonstrated how we fill in the blind spot with what our brains expect to be there.

Perception, however, is even more self-biased than that. Energy in the form we call light triggers signals in the rods and cones of the eye. The rods and cones are linked by ganglion cells, then other neurons that travel to a relay station in the brain stem called the lateral geniculate nucleus (Figure 2.2). Here, these neurons synapse with other sets of neurons that travel to the occipital lobe, the "seeing" part of the brain. The scientific belief was that stimuli in the retina were directly translated into impulses that were carried to the brain to be processed. However, studies of Manturana and Varela (1988) indicate that 80 percent of the electrical activity in the lateral geniculate body comes not from the eye but from the brain itself. The lateral geniculate body is not like a telephone switch that transmits signals without changing their content but is actually "translating" as it transmits signals, thus shaping the content of what we see.

The light we "see" is not the light from the world. There are no mirrors or fiber-optic pathways that transmit the light that enters the eye to the occipital lobes. The patterns of light we experience are released through changes in the rods and cones in the eye and invented within our visual system. In demonstration, we can provoke sensations of light by gently pressing on the closed eye. The cells of the eye have evolved to generate what we perceive as light when stimulated even if stimulated by pressure. The light we see is generated with our central nervous system. This is how we can experience light and color in our dreams.

Our learned expectations affect our perceptions in other ways. Look at Figure 2.3. In this example, because we are so accustomed to rectangular rooms, we see the two people as being of odd size rather than seeing the room as an unusual shape. In reality, the left side of the far wall is farther away from the observer, although the room has been arranged so that the eye sees a rectangle. When such illusions of perspective have been

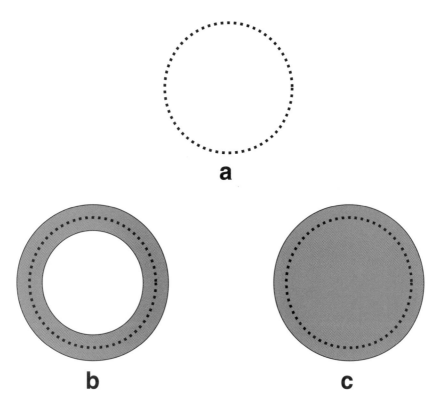

Figure 2.1. The blind spot. The visual system fills in the blind spot. In these experiments, a subject fixes on a point with one eye opened and one eye closed. (a) The location of the blind spot is identified and outlined. (b) A thick, colored ring of a size sufficient to stimulate the receptors around the margins of the blind spot is placed over the outline. (c) The subject reports seeing not a ring but a colored disk or dot.

shown to people who did not grow up with rectangular rooms (for example, an Australian aborigine) they have not perceived the paradox but have seen the odd-shaped room and the normal-sized people (Gregory 1986). Such experiments demonstrate that our past experiences affect our perception of the present.

To get another firsthand experience of how our learned expectations shape the world we experience, try the following simple experiment. Stand in front of a slightly "steamed" wet mirror after a shower and notice the size of your face. Draw an outline around your face. Your face looks to you like a *normal-size* face. Then step back to one side and look at the size of the outline on the mirror. The area outlined will be only half the size that the face had appeared to you.

Look at Figure 2.4. What do you see? Some people see faces, some people see goblets, and people who have seen this many times before see faces alternating with goblets. Our initial interpretations reveal and at the same time conceal what may be there. You see faces or goblets but not both simultaneously.

Experiments with placebos add another dimension to these examples. People who were undergoing tooth extraction were told that they would be intravenously given either demerol (a narcotic pain reliever) or saline (salt water) (Levine et al. 1978). They were asked to record their level of pain before and after the injections. About

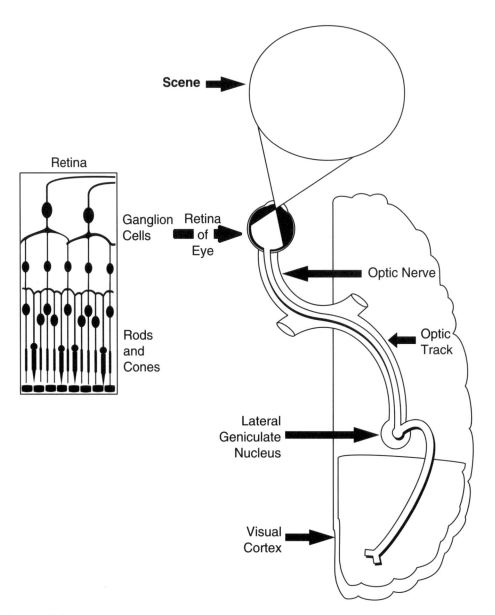

Figure 2.2. The visual system. Light entering the eye stimulates the rods and cones of the retina. Bioelectrical impulses are transmitted from the retina to the lateral geniculate nucleus (LGN) of the thalamus; here the neurons that entered the lateral geniculate body synapse with another set of neurons that travel to the visual cortex, the seeing part of the brain.

30 percent of the people who received saline reported a dramatic reduction in pain sensation. This is what is commonly known as the *placebo effect*. In itself, this was not a striking observation. What occurred next, however, was. The people who had experienced pain relief with the saline were then given naloxone, an antagonist to demerol, and their pain relief disappeared, that is, the level of pain returned to that

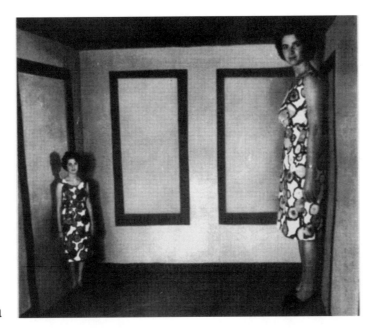

a

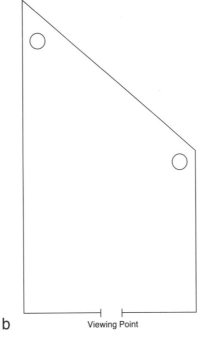

b   Viewing Point

Figure 2.3. Learned expectations affect our perceptions. (a) Accustomed to rectangular rooms, we see the two people as odd-sized rather than seeing the Ames's distorted room as an unusual shape. (b) In reality, the farther wall recedes from the observer to the left. The person on the left is actually distant, but the room's walls and windows and the painting of the walls are arranged so the eyes see a rectangular room.

Source: Eastern Daily Press (Norwich, England). Reprinted with permission.

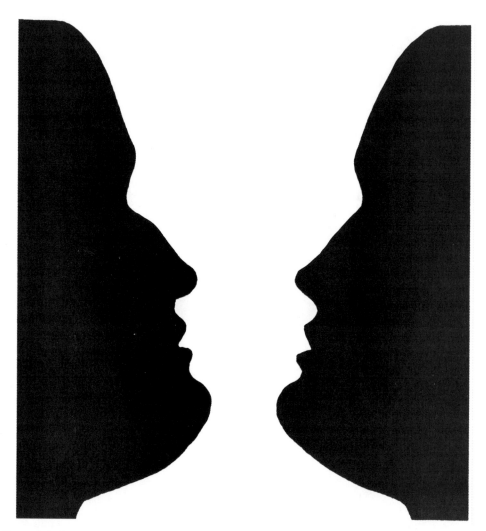

Figure 2.4. Perception. At first glance, you might see a goblet or two faces. If you continue to stare, you will see alternately one, then the other, but not both simultaneously.

prior to receiving the saline injection. Naloxone is also an antagonist to endogenous pain relievers such as endorphins. This experiment indicates that the subjects thinking that they were receiving a pain reliever actually altered the physical chemistry of their body, thus changing their experience of the pain. This alteration could be reversed by introducing another physical substance. Experiments such as these indicate that the way in which we physically experience the world is indeed affected by our thinking, our expectations, and our past conditioning.

These studies are presented to show how our predispositions constrain the ability of our primary senses to experience our world. A similar phenomenon also happens in our linguistic or narrative world as well, as is illustrated by the split brain (Gazzaniga 1978). A mammal's brain has two halves. Each receives sensory input from and affects motor

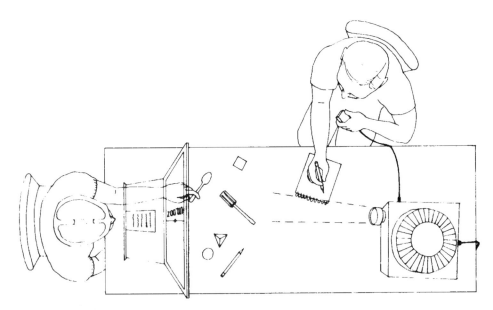

Figure 2.5. A tachistoscope simultaneously presents different images on the right and left sides of a screen while the subject concentrates on a dot in the center. The right half of the brain sees the image on the left side of the screen; the left side of the brain sees the image on the right side of the screen.

Source: Michael Gazzaniga and Joseph le Voux, *The Integrated Mind* (New York: Plenum Press, 1978). Used with permission.

control of the opposite side of the body. The halves are connected by the corpus callosum. Tachistoscope studies of patients in whom the corpus callosum has been split as part of epilepsy treatment (Gazzaniga 1978) have led to some interesting insights into human logic and behavior.

A tachistoscope simultaneously presents different images on the right and left sides of a screen while the subject concentrates on a dot in the center (Figure 2.5). The right half of the brain sees the image on the left side of the screen; the left side of the brain sees the image on the right side of the screen. Without a corpus callosum, there is no communication between the hemispheres. The experimenter requires the patient to point with the left hand to a picture or an object that matched what the right brain saw.

In one famous case, the tachistoscope presented a snowman and trees with snow on them on the left and a chicken's foot on the right (Figure 2.6). The patient's right brain saw the picture of snow and the left hand (right-brain function) picked a shovel. The left brain saw the chicken's foot. When a right-handed person was asked why he picked a shovel, he responded, "I saw a claw and I picked a shovel. You have to clean out the chicken shed with a shovel" (Gazzaniga 1978). Here, the left side of the brain had an explanation of why the right brain did what it had done, even though the left brain had no way of knowing why.

We are prone to storytelling, and we listen to our stories as though they are facts; for once we have a story, we usually do not reexamine the evidence for it, let alone the assumptions it is based on. The more important or more successful the story, the less we examine its underlying assumptions. We tend to interpret new data in terms of what we

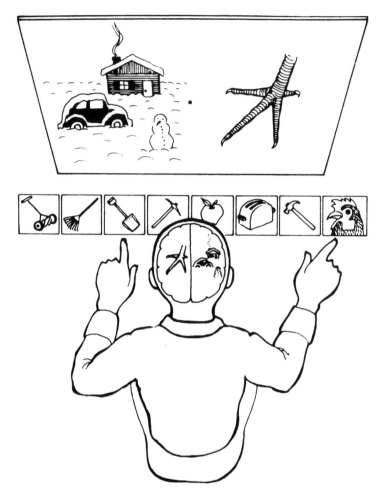

Figure 2.6. Split-brain experiment: a left-brain phenomenon: "The Interpreter." In one famous case, a tachistoscope presented in the left visual field a snowman and trees with snow on them and in the right visual field a chicken's foot. The right brain saw the picture of snow, and the left hand (right-brain function) picked a shovel. The left brain saw the chicken claw. When the right-handed subject was asked (i.e., left hemisphere was asked) why he picked the shovel, he responded, "I saw a claw and picked a shovel. You have to clean out the chicken shed with a shovel."

Source: Michael Gazzaniga, *The Integrated Mind* (New York: Plenum Press, 1978). Used with permission.

already know. We tend to fit the data to our story rather than fully attend to what we directly perceive and the potential implications for our worldviews.

Finally, all of the phenomena presented thus far happen before we are even aware of our world. Look at Figure 2.7. What do you see? Most people respond that the disk is off center or the figure is not balanced. The center, toward which the disk seems to strive, is not even an actual physical presence in the picture; yet, it is very much present in our perceptual experience. In our everyday lives, the effects of our conditioning are, for the most part, invisible to us. Our biases, preferences, and presuppositions are already incorpo-

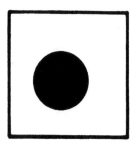

Figure 2.7. Disk in the rectangle. What do you immediately see? Most people respond that the disk is off center or the figure is not balanced. The center, toward which the disk seems to strive, is not even an actual physical presence in the picture; yet, it is very much present in our perceptual experience.

rated prior to our awareness of phenomena. It is only when we encounter a paradox or an anomaly that we have an opportunity to question our initial assumption.

When taken alone, the anomalies presented here remain isolated peculiarities and our basic assumptions go unquestioned. When juxtaposed, however, they begin to challenge the underlying assumption that we see reality without distortion.

These and other experiments are evidence that our past conditioning, current thinking, and expectations of the future shape the reality we perceive. Our past conditioning and current thinking become barriers to change. Are these claims too bold? To say that we may not see a world as it exists, that our thinking shapes our physical reality, may seem to fly in the face of common sense. However, in terms of evolutionary time, it was not that long ago that people believed and acted as though the world was flat because that is how it appeared to the eyes.

Common sense seems to tell us that knowledge eliminates ignorance. In other words, if we obtain more knowledge (more accurate representations), we will be better at solving problems. We do not see that many of our failures are not from the lack of knowledge, but from the failure and constraints of the knowledge that is already encoded in our brains.

Why present these studies in a text about QFD? First, to show how our past experiences and expectations of the future shape our perception of the world we see. Second, to show that these constraints are not just cultural, but constitutive to how the brain itself functions. Third, to build an awareness that these phenomenon limit key parts of designing quality.

If you were going to design a new product or service diligently, you would evaluate the capacities and limitations of the materials and parts you would use. Yet, we rarely consider the capacities and limitations presented by the fact that the human being is an essential component in many systems.

Finally, these ideas were presented to provide grounding for the statement that "We ordinarily dance with our internal maps of the world, not with the territory or world itself." There are different levels of "maps" or interpretations of the world available to us. To be more effective within the environment, we need to provoke a greater awareness of the external world. Our conceptual maps tend to be static pictures of the world and represent strategies that cling to what we see as certainty and avoid uncertainty. These maps are built upon assumptions, some so successful we have forgotten they were originally assumptions. In other words, we need to access more of the light that strikes the retina and less of the "light" that we generate in the lateral geniculate body and visual cortex to shift our attention to perceptions arising from the environment and away from our concepts, our beliefs. We need data and motivation to overcome our natural homeostatic tendencies, our *psychological inertia.*

We use the term *inertia* in the same sense as is used in physics. That is, a body in motion tends to stay in motion or a body at rest tends to stay at rest unless acted on by an outside force. If you roll a ball along the floor, it will, until acted on by outside forces such as the friction on the floor or a wall, continue rolling in the direction it is going. The same is true of systems. Systems in motion tend to remain in motion in the direction they are moving until acted on by other forces. This is true of an individual cell, an individual human being, or social organizations. A difference between an inanimate object such as a ball and a living organization, however, is that relatively low energy level stimuli that may have little or no effect on an inanimate object can produce change in the function of the living system.

In psychological and organizational management, the term *resistance* is applied when we as leaders or managers introduce a request for change but the system continues in the direction it was going. In the text, we prefer to use the term *psychological inertia.* Resistance implies an us-and-them relationship; we have applied the "right stimulus"; and they are resisting the change. Psychological inertia is more emotionally neutral. It includes the possibility that the outside stimulus or force we as managers have brought to bear is insufficient to alter homeostatic or inertial stability of the system.

Earlier, we suggested a fundamental premise to Western science, and our common-sense view of reality includes realism, separateness, and inductive prediction. We then presented some visual experiments that challenged assumptions of realism. This is the essence of scientific method:

1. Form hypothesis—here, that we see a world without distortion.

2. Do experiments to test principles that should be consistent with the hypothesis.

3. Do the experiments, collect data, and compare the data to the hypothesis.

4. Accept, reject, or modify the hypothesis.

When the preceding figures and experiments are taken separately, they can be seen as peculiar anomalies or paradoxes. When taken together, these examples indicate that our experience of the present is influenced by past experiences. They also challenge the assumption that we see reality without distortion. We interpret our world with the structure and function of the nervous system, and our past affects how we envision the present and the future. There are many examples of this in medicine, for example, phantom pain and referred pain. If we experienced a world without distortion, how could a person experience pain in a limb no longer there? Phantom pain, that is, pain in an extremity that has been amputated, arises with the body's learned representation of the limb from past experience.

We are interpreters of our world. Our reality is an aggregate of perceptions from our primary senses, physical sensations, and moods and emotions perceived as arising from our bodies and the thoughts and conversations going on in our heads. We could use an analogy of watching a TV with the following channels:

1. Language channel: stories, narratives, conceptual maps of a world

2. Sensory channel: the data we generated from our primary senses—sights, sounds, touch, taste, and smell

3. Emotional channel: moods, emotions, and the inner sensations these generate

As seen with the Ames's room, our perceptual maps are shaped by our past experience. The past filters and molds how we expect the world to show up. These visual exercises, like the early steps of QFD, were designed to capture and to interpret data for the environmental world to stimulate a reevaluation of conceptual maps, presuppositions, and beliefs to shift the actions that flow from these. Ideally, an individual, a team, or an organization would then, based upon the data captured for the environment, alter their narratives and conceptual maps. This is the core process in the scientific method.

This is how scientific experimentation is supposed to be carried out in the laboratory setting. In practice, however, we have an emotional charge linked to our conceptual maps, and this emotional charge constrains or accelerates our ability to adapt to change. The initial steps in QFD are designed to capture and rank data from the environment (the sensory channel). The correlation matrices used in subsequent steps can be viewed as a set of tools to hold before us what was perceived as important (ranked data from the sensory channel) even if it challenges sacred assumptions (the language/conceptual channel) and to catalyze (reduce) the inertial forces to overcome the charged moods and emotions (the emotional channel).

The early tools of QFD assume that we, by and large, have been conditioned by our past experiences and seek to transcend this conditioning by attending to stimuli that are triggered by customers and environments to identify what is meaningful to customers and potential customers, that is, to listen to the voice of the customer. This is the essence of the initial step in the QFD process. Subsequent steps are designed to keep attention on what is meaningful to customers before us to overcome our psychological inertia as we design processes and systems to deliver products and services that result in meaning.

ALGORITHMS: STRUCTURED PROCESSES

Our maps are unevenly biased by our experiences. Studies of how medical decisions are made by physicians indicate that a limited number of "great successes" and "disastrous failures" are weighted disproportionately high relative to a large number of "reasonably good outcomes" in daily decision-making processes. Recent successes and failures weigh more heavily than distant experiences. These factors account for some of the variation in healthcare. Variations in practice patterns of different physicians in the same context and variation by the same physician from case to case have also been well documented.

Einhorn (1972) compared physicians' clinical judgment to an actuarial judgment (an algorithm). Three highly trained pathologists were required to predict survival time following the initial diagnosis of Hodgkin's disease, a form of cancer. Each reviewed initial biopsy slides used to make the diagnosis in 193 cases selected from a large metropolitan hospital. All patients in the study had subsequently died, providing an observable end point for length of survival. Each pathologist was asked to identify nine histological characteristics used in standard practice to determine the severity of the disease and then rate each of these characteristics on a five-point scale of severity. The pathologists were then asked, based on their evaluations of these characteristics and their experience, to estimate the survival time based on the severity of the disease. The higher the severity of the disease, the shorter the survival time. Correlation coefficients for the three pathologists and actual outcome were 0.00, +0.11, and –0.14. In contrast, an algorithmic actuarial formula based on the same nine histological characteristics that the pathologists ranked achieved a mean correlation of –0.30.

Found 51 studies comparing human judgment to mechanical or algorithmic tools
In 33, actuarial methods significantly better than human judgment (p>0.05)
In 17, actuarial methods better than human judgment but not at p>0.05 level
In one, human judgment significantly better (p>0.05)

Figure 2.8. Algorithms versus usual human judgment. Meehl (1965) collected 51 studies comparing human judgment to mechanical or algorithmic tools.

Meehl (1965) collected 51 studies comparing human judgment to mechanical methods such as actuarial formulas or algorithms (Figure 2.8). In 33 studies, the actuarial method was significantly better than human judgment (P > 0.050). In 17 cases, the actuarial method was not better, but the difference was not statistically significant. In one case, the human judgment was better.

The figures and the discussion of figures presented in this chapter are included to make present biases and presuppositions in our everyday perceptual/conceptual mechanisms. The data of Einhorn and Meehl are included to make present limitations in our categorizing and decision-making habits. Our common-sense notions suggest that we make decisions by

1. Identifying a set of options

2. Identifying ways of evaluating these options

3. Weighting each evaluation/dimension

4. Doing the weighting

5. Picking the option with the highest weight

However, Soelberg (1967) studied how students at MIT chose their jobs upon graduation to prove the foregoing as a hypothesis. The results showed that, instead, students made "gut choices" and the preceding steps were actually carried out after the fact to support their choices.

Data of de Groot (1946), who studied chess masters; data of Kahneman and Teversky (1982), who studied people in the laboratory setting; and data of Klein and colleagues (1999), who studied firefighters and military personnel, suggest we use a simulation heuristic to make most decisions. That is, most of us construct an imaginary model based on past experiences and visualize how it works. Klein and colleagues suggest that if the model was a machine it would have a maximum size of three moving parts (i.e., three interrelated variables) and its function would be limited to six steps or transition states.

In designing a machine, we would certainly want to consider the strengths and weaknesses (i.e., the tolerances) of its parts. Yet, many organizations do not do so when designing processes. They take for granted a key part, the human being.

A surgeon would not go in to perform a complex medical procedure without the appropriate tools. A hospital administrator would not take on a large home-improvement project without appropriate tools. Yet, both hospital management and medical staffs routinely "wing it" without tools when it comes to designing and redesigning complex services and care issues. In the case example and subsequent discussions, we will show how the tools and the algorithm of QFD can be used to compare and rank 60 demanded qualities by customers and how a 20 item by 20 item matrix can be used to evaluate and rank the 400 different interactions between these items.

Processes and algorithms can be used as strategies to overcome our psychological inertia and cultural biases, to listen to customers, and to translate the customer's voice into organizational performance measures, functions, and tasks. This is the heart of QFD. In the absence of such practices, we, like the three pathologists, will not be consistently successful. In today's world, the continued success of an organization is related to its ability to overcome the constraints of the past—its ability to change.

CHANGE IS A JOURNEY, NOT AN EVENT

Success in today's rapidly changing environment is almost synonymous with the capacity to change. Change is not easy. Several studies have suggested that more than two-thirds of change projects fail to produce their anticipated results. Why?

Change is an ongoing process and not a single event. Organizations, whether cells or businesses, cannot introduce a new class of output (functions) unless they alter their underlying structure (Fritz, 1996). The process of change for individuals, as well as organizations, follows a change pattern similar to an enzymatic reaction in a simple cell. We refer to this pattern of change in the cell as an archetype for the journey of change. An enzymatic change can be plotted as a change in energy or work over time (Figure 2.9). Point 1 in the figure is the current state (Compounds A and B), and Point 4 is the target state (Compound C). In between are an early transition phase (Point 2) and a late transition phase (Point 3). Both Points 2 and 3 embody a higher degree of energy, complexity, and tension than either the current or target states. In other words, transition states are unstable and seek resolution by moving toward lesser states of complexity.

Most transitional encounters that reach Point 2 follow the path of least resistance and revert back to Point 1. No net change occurs. If the process does reach Point 3, the instability is again resolved by following the path of least resistance—this time by releasing energy and forming the new structure (Compound C). Energy is required to successfully transform Compounds A and B into Compound C. Biological catalysts, such as enzymes, reduce the amount of energy and work required to achieve successful change.

When we embark on either a personal or organizational journey of change (moving toward Point 2), we have to give up the comforts and safety of the known before the promises and rewards of the new are available to us. Our attention becomes trapped by what we perceive as losses and our fears of an uncertain future. These uncertainties and perceived losses trigger powerful emotions in both individuals and organizations similar to those described by Elizabeth Kübler-Ross (1997) for the process of death and dying: denial, anger, yes but, depression, and acceptance. Denial, anger, compromise, resignation, and hopelessness (depression) are powerful inhibitors to individual and organizational change. Like the disk that already appears off center, our ordinary everyday view of the world shows up to us already colored and shaped by our moods, emotions, and judgments. The latter contribute to the psychological inertia and homeostatic mechanisms that keep us bound to our "sacred" presuppositions, our beliefs.

Many journeys of change stop at Point 2, and, over time, behavior and processes revert back to the comfortable old ways, Point 1. Some processes of change become stuck in a more complex state, requiring more work and energy to maintain but never realizing the promising potentials. Some organizations cycle between Points 1 and 2. Many organizations embark on and are committed to their journeys, but they fail to alter

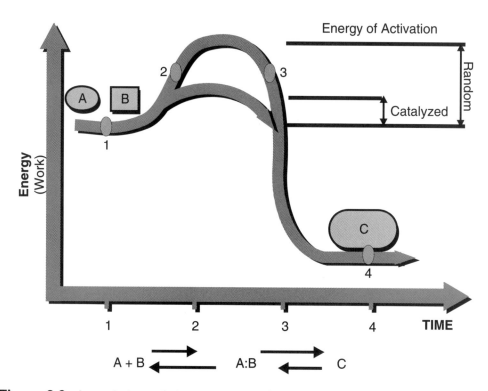

Figure 2.9. An archetype of change: enzymatic workflow. An enzymatic reaction is plotted as the change in energy (vertical axis) over a period of time (horizontal axis). Initially, increase in the energy of the system—energy of activation—is required to overcome the steady state inertia before the process can move from a state of higher energy to lower energy. Four points in time along this journey can be identified; Point 1, the initial state; Point 2, early transition state; Point 3, late transition state; and Point 4, target or destination.

their structure to support change. Either they fail to provide the tools and training to change skills or they fail to align rewards and consequences to change human behavior.

Our, deep-seated and long-standing habits still shape our perceptions and actions in ways of which we are unaware. Thinking paternalistically, making the customer wrong, and narrowly focusing on events have been historical barriers to incorporating the voice of the customer into the design of healthcare services. The TQM movement shifted awareness from events to processes. QFD will shift some of the attention from individual processes (the parts) to designing system structures and relationships (the whole) so that processes are linked to customers. QFD is a set of connected practices that are like a series of enzymatic reactions. When employed, these practices link us with stimuli from the environment, lower barriers and resistance to change, and dramatically improve success rates.

Chapter 3

The Cell: A Model
for an Organization

Upon completion of this chapter, you will have a sense of:

- A fundamental source or root cause for breakdowns in our social organizations

- How organizations that adapt and survive have healthy internal structures (anatomy); have functional internal patterns of relationships (physiology); generate and exchange value (biochemistry); and are intimately coupled to their environment (ecology)

- How our biology predisposes us to cling to past successes and thus to live past-based futures

- A map of the exchange of value, and the exchange of value, that is the glue that holds our social units together

The last chapter reviewed some of the barriers to healthcare organizations for incorporating the voice of the customer. Before actually getting into QFD as a process, this chapter uses distinctions learned in high-school biology to present a high-level schema for the underlying design of one of the most successful knowledge-based, process-focused organizations on the planet. This narrative and image provide a framework upon which to interpret key distinctions and relationships in QFD.

CRITICAL CHALLENGES

All social organizations, be they communities or businesses, face three critical challenges:

- Aligning around a common purpose, then agreeing upon and delivering value in that environment

- Managing internal specialization (differentiation) while maintaining organizational alignment (integration)

- Adapting to a rapidly changing environment

Consider the problem of world hunger. There is more than enough food produced on the planet to prevent people from dying of starvation, yet starvation continues to be a problem in many parts of the world. Periodically, we are confronted by pictures of young children malnourished and dying. There is an effort to transport the food from areas of plenty to areas of scarcity. Yet, local political friction often prevents distribution of the food. Somalia is just one example. This is the problem created when all participants are not aligned around a common purpose, that is, they are not in agreement as to what is important.

No one reading this text would let the person who lives next door to them starve to death. Yet, we go about our day-to-day lives as people starve in lands apart from us. This is the problem of separation. In the system that includes world hunger, we are a differentiated part of a larger integrated whole. Our physical bodies have evolved over millions of years to respond to what is immediately before us. We are predisposed to focus on the short-term, quick fixes for the issues before us and de-emphasize long-term and complex problems. When the media flashes images of starving children, we open our pocketbooks or react in some other appropriate manner. When the media no longer focuses on world hunger, we become separated from the issue. The problem is out of sight and out of mind, and we move on to something else.

Even if we remain attentive and committed to working on world hunger, the sheer scope of the problem, the paucity of reinforcing and nurturing feedback for our actions, and the abundance of negative feedback that our actions do not really make a difference predispose us to resignation and resentment. The latter are very disempowering emotions. These three problems are major sources (root causes) of many of the personal and organizational breakdowns:

- Lack of agreement about what is important

- Separation or fragmentation that allows us to focus on parts of the system rather than the whole

- The lack of immediate reinforcing feedback to initiate and reinforce change efforts

When what is important is seen as clear and urgent, most established organizations respond effectively. Examples would be a *code blue,* a code trauma in an emergency room, and other "firefighting" activities in hospitals. These are examples where what is important is clear, roles are defined, and feedback is immediate. In the absence of such a unifying, clear, and urgent sense of what is important, each person, department, and division tends to focus on what is immediately before them. In a busy hospital setting, the task that is triaged to a lower level of priority often does not get the attention it requires even though it may alleviate acute crises in the long run. In many hospitals, the basic feedback strategies—such as chart audits for quality—are so delayed and separate from day-to-day, hands-on care that the information often has little impact on day-to-day activities.

CELLS AS MODELS

Our linguistic and conceptual capacities to plan and coordinate future actions give us the capacity to design systems that take advantage of our strengths and compensate for our weaknesses in order to avoid the pitfalls of human nature. QFD, at its core, is about design—designing processes and systems to meet the challenges just discussed. Our common-sense notion is that design is about putting parts together to generate a larger whole. However, neither the cells in our bodies nor our bodies as a whole result from putting parts together. In nature, the whole precedes the parts and complexity derives from a series of actions that unfold within the whole. Each of us started from a single cell—a whole that divided into two parts, which divided into four, and so on. The problem of differentiation and integration is solved naturally by enfolding complexity into a whole, not vice versa.

We use the cell as a model of a self-organizing and self-regulating system—a model of a whole and its parts. Cells have survived two billion years and are still going strong. As whole systems, cells have structure, internal relationships, capacity for action, and sets of relationships with their environment.

Structure: Anatomy

Cells are knowledge-based organisms. *Knowledge,* as defined here, is the capacity to generate actions based on past experience. In other words, knowledge is know-how. Cells store, recall, and deploy knowledge to generate effective actions. The knowledge stored in DNA is transcribed to RNA and then translated in proteins. Proteins as enzymes catalyze actions, converting resources (possibilities) into product (results) (Figure 3.1).

DNA encodes the knowledge of what has worked in the past. RNA is a template for future structures and future action. This juxtaposition of the future projected ahead of the present generates direction as it calls forth, informs, and shapes the actions that unfold in the present (Figure 3.1). DNA also encodes what actions will be preferentially catalyzed and allowed within the organization. By generating direction and setting boundaries for actions, DNA shapes the nature of the cell, which encompasses the very nature of the whole—be it lion or lamb.

This simple pattern of future juxtaposed ahead of the present as a way to generate direction and to align and order actions in the present is repeated throughout all levels of living entities, from cells to bodies and from bodies to social units (including business organizations). This pattern is so basic to all levels of our existence that it is transparent to us.

Reach for an object in front of you. How did you do that? Although some of us have a story about what happened, we really do not know. Capacities to act and create extend far beyond our current understanding of action and creativity. When you reach for that object (a target), a template of the future is juxtaposed ahead of your stored capacity to generate actions incorporated during past experience. This juxtaposition generates and shapes the actions that unfold in the present as you reach for the target.

As human beings, our memories of the past are transcribed ahead of us, generating our expectations. Expectations, in turn, guide our actions in the present. The projection of visions for the future also generates direction and purpose for our social organizations. The future satisfaction of the customer/patient can be deployed to shape organizational structure and behavior.

Internal Patterns of Relationships: Physiology

Cells have sets of interrelationships. Enzymes, the structural basis for actions in the present, become linked to form processes. Interconnected processes work as units to transform resources into more valued products. The results of these actions feed back to

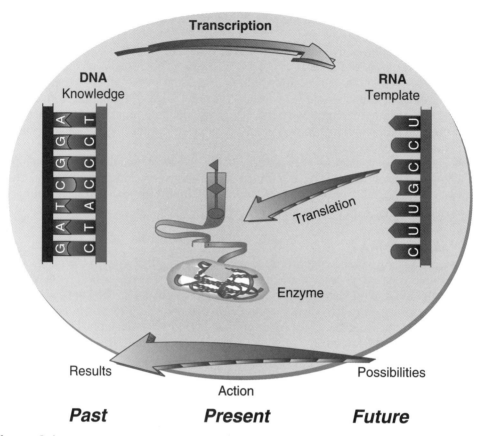

Figure 3.1. The cell as a temporal organization. Knowledge of what occurred in the past is stored in DNA. The knowledge in DNA is transcribed into RNA, a template of a future action. The information in RNA is, in turn, translated into a structure, an enzyme. Enzymes catalyze the conversion of possibilities into results.

inform the parts (enzymes, processes, and genetic leadership) and automatically adjust actions as the system pursues its targets (Figure 3.2).

In biological systems, there are two major types of feedback: those that are symmetrical or reinforcing (where increasing input increases output) and those that are complementary or balancing (where increasing input decreases or inhibits output). The relationships of input to output are typically nonlinear. Such feedback systems are very sensitive to subtle changes in key variables. Small shifts in key variables can produce large shifts in the response of the entire system. In this way, small changes in the sequences of symmetrical and complementary processes are able to balance each other and self-regulate cellular processes.

As your arm moves when you reach for an object, sensors in the muscles and joints provide information about the arm's position in space to the brain, which is then able to coordinate action so that you are able to reach the target. The mesh of interconnected processes and feedback from actions modifies those actions, generating a self-regulating,

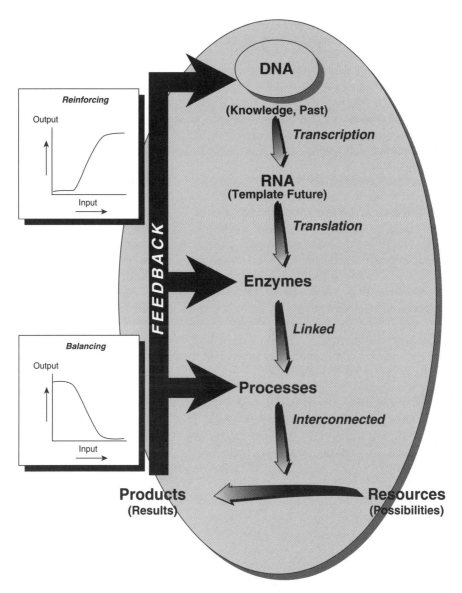

Figure 3.2. Interconnected processes and feedback. Enzymes become linked into interconnected processes. The results of these processes convert resources into products. The products result in feedback organizing the activity of enzymes, processes, and the genetic leadership of the cell.

self-organizing whole. This network of feedback and automatic adjustments is the basis for the phenomenon we call homeostasis.

Generation and Exchange of Value: Biochemistry

At some point billions of years ago, the parts of the cell joined together to form larger wholes, generating more value than the parts could generate alone. The flow and exchange of value between the parts are the glue that holds the parts together to form the whole. Biochemistry maps the generation and exchange of value within the cell as the flow of energy.

There is no master gene in the cell, nor is there a master cell in the body. Processes are interconnected. For example, high-energy ATP links the processes of consumption and production. The energy released in converting glucose to carbon dioxide and water is captured in high-energy ATP, which can then be used to generate proteins, muscle actions, and so on, important to the function of the organization. When these linkages become uncoupled and production and consumption become unbalanced, diseases occur.

External Patterns of Relationships: Ecology

The individual parts of living organisms are continuously sensitive to the environment for signals, which are then disseminated throughout the whole body. The interplay of internal feedback and environmental signals generates minute-to-minute adjustments in enzymes and processes, while it also informs and shapes actions at the genetic level. Genetic activity, in turn, either adjusts targets or calls forth entirely new targets. New targets generate new structures that catalyze new actions (Figure 3.3). This self-organizing system seeks stability but is simultaneously stimulated toward change by an everchanging environment.

When you reach for an object, the target (future state) is juxtaposed ahead of your capacity to act (knowledge accumulated from past experience). This juxtaposition sets a direction and shapes the action that unfolds in the present. As your arm moves, sensors in the muscles and joints generate internal feedback that adjusts the activity of the muscles. Your eyes constantly capture signals from the environment. If the object moves, these signals trigger an adjustment in the target and the action of the arm. In the language of systems, thinking targets are feed-forward loops and measures of the results are the unfolding feedback loops. Together, the feed-forward and feedback loops shape actions that unfold in the present (Figure 3.4).

This same fundamental pattern shapes and orders our social bodies, including business organizations (Figure 3.5). Leaders transcribe templates of the future—visions, vivid images, and powerful narratives. As in the cell, visions of the future are juxtaposed ahead of the organization's stored capacity for action accumulated through past experiences. The relationship between this image of the future and knowledge of the past generates dynamic tension and sets direction and purpose. This purpose, guided by established cultural principles, sets the boundaries of acceptable actions. Purpose and principles for action generate the structure of the organization (the deep-skeletal foundation) and the boundaries for action. Just as the DNA of the single-celled embryo contains the nature of the mature organism, the purpose and principles for valued actions (virtue and values) set the identity and nature of our social organizations.

Within this broad framework, leaders and managers also design and communicate more refined templates for actions with greater differentiation; these are business and management strategies. These templates generate spatial/temporal maps that give identity to the whole and guide the actions of the parts. The templates inform and shape the unfolding of structures, then support the differentiated actions necessary to create the whole. These actions are integrated through feedback to both the parts and the whole.

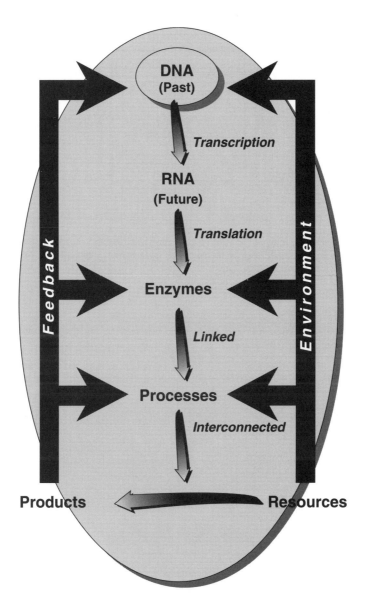

Figure 3.3. Cells are constantly capturing signals from the environment. These signals are disseminated throughout the organization to processes, individual enzymes, and the genetic leadership of the cell.

CHANGE

The cell's capacity to change its function is limited by its structure. When living organizations attempt to perform beyond their structural capacity, they generate consequences that feed back and inhibit the organization's capacity to perform. For example, a sprinter can only run at a very fast pace over a short distance because muscles generate lactic acid at high speeds, inhibiting their capacity to work. Before the sprinter can go faster

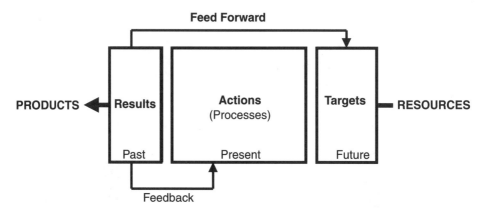

Figure 3.4. A system diagram. The results of past action—learning—become targets for the future. These targets call forth actions that, in turn, generate results. The results provide feedback that modifies actions.

or longer, he or she must train. The repetitive activity of training is an outside demand, a stimulus to the muscles to change their enzymatic structure to meet an environmental challenge.

Living organizations change in response to a changing environment in three broad ways:

- Minute-to-minute adaptations occur through the mesh of interconnections and feedback that we call homeostasis.

- Stimuli from the environment overwhelm the status quo, and cells refer to their store of past experiences to find an effective response.

  Both of these reactions are derived from past successes and keep the organization's future tied to its past.

- Environmental change goes beyond anything experienced in the past, forcing a shift to a future based on possibility instead of experience. A new class of actions must be designed for this target, or the organization will perish. As they say in environmental science, "Adapt or die."

In most of the body cells, the time from the appearance of a perturbation that signals a need for change at the surface of the cell (e.g., a estrogen) until the appearance of a valued result is 60 to 90 minutes (Figure 3.6). The time from the appearance of RNA in the body of the cell (the target) to the appearance of a valued product is only one to two minutes. At least 95 percent of the cell's response time is focused on processing the implications of signals and then designing and transcribing strategic responses.

We now have a view of the living entity, be it body cell or business organization. Our social organizations are dynamic and living extensions of our being. Living entities are self-enclosing, self-organizing wholes with a natural tendency to live a future based on the past. Left to our own devices, our natural tendency is to recreate our past successes over and over again. It is only through interactions with our environment that we can transcend the limits of our past.

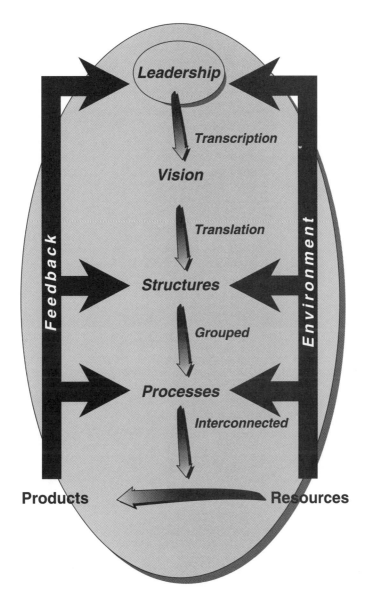

Figure 3.5. The human social organization as a living system. The organization's leadership transcribes visions—targets of future state—into structures to support the activities and processes necessary to convert necessary resources into products to achieve the vision. The results of the actions feed back to the organization. Dynamic organizations also constantly capture information from the environment.

This cellular model embodies two cycles. In one, targets from the past are transcribed and translated into future targets that shape our actions as they unfold in the present. This is the source of our past-based futures. Organizations that remain trapped within scenarios of the future that are based on past successes cannot adapt to rapidly changing environments. In the second cycle, possibilities for new futures are triggered

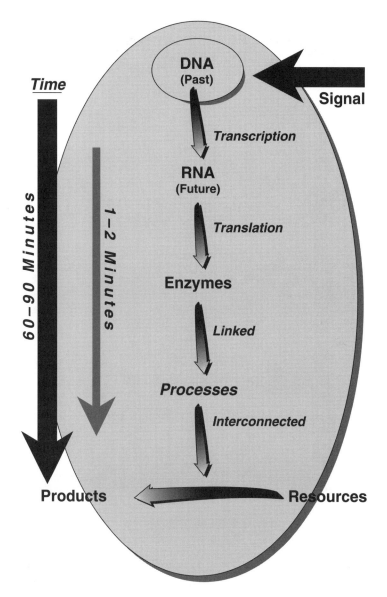

Figure 3.6. Processing stimuli from the environment. The time from when a signal reaches a cell—for example, the hormone estrogen on a uterine cell—to the time of identifying products the hormone triggers in the cytoplasm or body of the cell is approximately 60 to 90 minutes. The time from the appearance of the RNA target in the cytoplasm to the appearance of the product is one to two minutes.

by the environment. However, organizations that chase every new environment stimulus risk losing their connection to past successes. Their core competencies become fragmented and feeble. A balance is needed. QFD, a set of tools that link customer wants and needs (environmental stimuli) to core competencies (past successes), provides the balance.

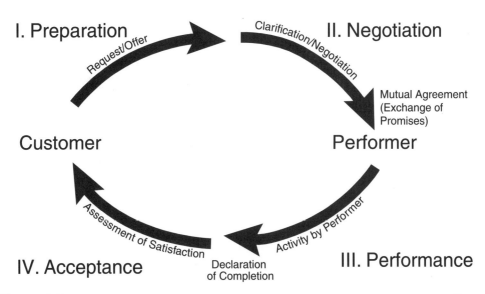

Figure 3.7. ActionWorkflow®. Our social interactions are exchange reactions. They begin by a request from a customer or an offer from a provider (preparation phase). The customer or provider may require clarification, and this negotiation phase ends with the mutual agreement or mutual exchange of promises (negotiation phase). The performer then carries out the work—the performance phase—and declares the performance complete. The customer then has an assessment of satisfaction or dissatisfaction (satisfaction phase).

Source: Modified from R. Dunham, "Business Design Technology; Software Development for Customer Satisfaction," *Proceedings of the 24th Annual Hawaii International Conference on Systems Sciences* 3(1991):792. Reprinted with permission, Action Technologies, Alameda, Calif.

MAPPING OUR SOCIAL WORLDS

Like the cells in our body, at some point in our history, human beings joined together to form larger organizations that were capable of generating greater value. Social interactions are about both the generation of value and the exchange of that value. Like the high-energy ATP that connects the processes of consumption and production in the cell, commitments (promises and requests) interconnect and coordinate the generation (production) and exchange (consumption) of value in our social bodies.

Just as the flow of energy and information at a quantum level becomes manifest at the human level of physical experience, the flow of requests and promises in human interactions forms a network that creates the structure of our social organizations. The assessment of user satisfaction or dissatisfaction underlies the exchange of value in our social world. These phenomena can be mapped in the same way that we map the biochemistry of the cell.

Consider the simple task of going to a coffee shop for a cup of coffee (Figure 3.7). The exchange interaction is as follows:

- Phase I, preparation: A customer makes a request of the provider.

- Phase II, negotiation: There is clarification and negotiation about the type of coffee that is wanted.

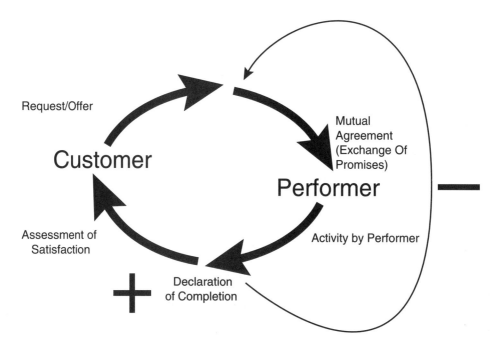

Figure 3.8. Feedback. ActionWorkflow® can be used to map out the processes as well as the reinforcing (positive) and balancing (negative) feedback within those processes.

- Phase III, performance: Certain actions are performed leading to a completed transaction; a cup of coffee is served.

- Phase IV, acceptance: The customer indicates acceptance of the transaction by making payment. The customer is either satisfied or dissatisfied with the product or service and, based on this assessment, will or will not return to the shop.

ActionWorkflow® (Dunham 1991; ActionWorkflow®) can be used to map out the processes as well as the reinforcing (positive) and balancing (negative) feedback within these processes (Figure 3.8). For example, the customer's perceptions and actions upon the "declaration of completion" by the provider (end of performance, phase III) provide reinforcing or inhibiting feedback. If the customer is satisfied, the satisfaction reinforces the actions within the cycle. If the customer is not satisfied, he or she may say so, which inhibits the cycle and may stimulate renegotiation. "This cup of coffee is cold. I want . . ." will initiate another loop until customer satisfaction is achieved.

The exchange of value captured by this four-phase cycle is the glue that holds our everyday social interactions together. Healthcare is a series of chain handoff processes that create value for customers. The efficiency of chain handoff processes can be increased by shortening their length, increasing their throughput or decreasing variations across the handoff through feed-forward and feedback mechanisms.

The network of commitments that underlie chain handoff processes can be mapped using ActionWorkflow® (Figure 3.7) as a business process tool (Chaplin 1996). The challenge facing healthcare organizations is to identify what will produce customer satisfaction and then deploy the skills and competencies of the organization in networks of commitment that generate the action necessary to produce conditions of satisfaction. QFD is a set of tools that deploy processes to do just that. QFD begins by distinguishing what is required to generate customer satisfaction, then defines what actions need to be performed to create those conditions in an efficient and reliable manner.

In the next chapter, we will present an overview of QFD as a set of tools that address the challenges presented to all organizations, from cell to business:

- What are the organization's targets?

- What performance measures for the organization's actions are going to be used as feedback to navigate and define conditions that will indicate when the targets have been satisfactorily delivered?

- How is the organization going to use these measures to align actions with organizational rewards and consequences to design and implement self-organizing and self-regulating systems?

- How is the organization going to capture information from the environment and incorporate this information into its organizational structures and functions?

The QFD process begins by defining what conditions are necessary to produce customer assessments of satisfaction (acceptance phase, Figure 3.7) and identifying the actions that need to be performed to provide these conditions (performance phase, Figure 3.7).

QFD matches the voice of the customer to the performance of the organization. It promotes the design of products and services that generate value from the customer's perspective. The generation of value and the exchange of value between an organization and its customers are the lifeblood of the organization.

Like cells, where more than 95 percent of response time involves capturing and processing the implications of environmental perturbations, the key focus in a QFD process is capturing information from the environment in order to distinguish and design specific targets and structures for action. Reaching Point 4 on the archetypal journey of change (see Figure 2.9) requires setting targets based on customer importance. Identifying key functions, critical tasks, and feedback measures integrates and focuses us on what is important in the present and catalyzes the shift from Point 2 to Point 3. Once these structures are in place, actions flow from the resulting processes to Point 4 as naturally as breath does from a body.

We now have the necessary tools for organizational diagnosis:

1. The model of the cell can be used as a lens to distinguish and diagnose healthy and unhealthy structures and sets of relationships and to value exchanging mechanisms and the ecology of organizational processes.

2. The example of our inability to alleviate world hunger illustrates three breakdown points: (1) definition of and agreement on what is important, (2) a biological predisposition to respond to the more immediate tasks and discount long-term consequences, and (3) resignation and resentment that result from inadequate or delayed feedback.

3. ActionWorkflow® is a diagnostic map to identify breakdowns in the exchange of value between customers and performers, whether the breakdown is within the organization or between the organization and its environment.

These three tools can be used to identify at a very fundamental level the breakdown of social units within an organization. We now return to QFD to design treatment or intervention strategies, creating more healthy and healing spaces for the problems that ail social units.

Chapter 4

Overview of the Tool Set:
A Hospital-Based Case Study

Upon completion of this chapter, you will have:

- An introductory overview of a case

- An acquaintance with some of the tools used in comprehensive QFD

In chapter 1, we briefly reviewed key distinctions of QFD as a process (see Figure 1.5 and Figure 1.6). While still working at a conceptual level, we now provide more details, with the goal of generating a sense of the algorithm or process that QFD embodies. The added detail is used to show how the different steps are linked, how highly weighted customer demands are identified, and how these demands are implemented in day-to-day tasks. If chapter 1 was a 10,000-foot view, the initial section of this chapter is the 1000-foot level. The remainder of the chapter is more detailed and introduces some of the tools and steps in QFD, a 500-foot view. Part 2 of the text is a ground-level view, giving details of how data is captured from the environment, the step-by-step process that generates relationship matrices, and the output of analyses.

The following detailed overview is given to provide a structure for understanding the QFD tools as they are introduced in the workbook section. This case study has been simplified to emphasize distinctions important to QFD as a set of structures and relationships. The example is taken from a QFD project at a rehabilitation hospital that provides comprehensive medical and/or legal evaluations for people with complex and catastrophic injuries or illnesses. After redesigning the evaluation process, the organization experienced a twofold rise in the rate of referrals for the service. These services are low in volume, complex, provider intensive, and expensive. Each patient is different and thus requires a somewhat unique and extensive evaluation.

A typical evaluation includes physical capacity assessments and radiological tests such as computerized axial tomography (CAT) scans, magnetic resonance imaging (MRI), and bone scans. The evaluations are conducted by four to eight physicians from different specialties. Two to three specialty-related therapy evaluations are also performed. In addition, the process requires the work of 10 to 25 other staff members, including people from nursing, technical support, and administrative support. These activities may be coordinated between as many as 10 different business organizations, with complex radiological testing and physician evaluations supplied by separate business entities. Almost all requests for this service come from workers' compensations insurers. The goal of the QFD project was to increase the volume of referrals for the service.

There are ongoing discussions within the healthcare industry about who is the primary customer for healthcare services. We personally are pretty clear about that. It is "we the people," the people who need the services, individuals whether healthy or ill, and the communities they live in. From the perspective of a healthcare-delivery organization, however, there are a variety of customer segments and stakeholders whose behaviors influence the quality and viability of any particular service. As you will see in Part 2, the model of QFD we are presenting includes a set of tools to identify customer segments and stakeholders and what is important to each. For a hospital, stakeholders include patients, physicians, staff, insurers, employers, regulatory agencies, and so on. The tools of QFD and the purpose of the QFD project identify who the primary customers and stakeholders are for that particular project. As already mentioned, the goal of the QFD team in the case example was to increase the volume of referrals for the service. Meeting the service needs of the insurer was identified as having the highest probability of accomplishing the goal. For other services and projects, the major customer segment might be the patient, the physicians who refer patients, a regulatory agency, a neighborhood, a community or so on. As you will see in Part 2, many hospital services must satisfy all simultaneously—patient, referring and attending physicians, and regulatory agencies.

CASE OVERVIEW: THE OUTPUT (1000-FOOT VIEW)

The project team embraced the customer-driven philosophy of QFD. Their first step was to identify customer segments and to select the key segments. The team selected the insurers as their primary customer group. After identification of the customer segment, the QFD team developed its understanding of the user by meeting with and observing a representative sample in the user's environment. The team asked why and how the sample group used the organization's services. After this information was gathered, the team translated the customers' demanded qualities into performance measures and set targets for each of those performance measures.

In this way, the team developed an understanding of how the service fits into the customer's overall process and identified 80 items that were important to those customers. Working with a small group of customers and the tools of QFD, these items were ranked in order of most to least importance by the customers themselves. The eight most highly ranked items were chosen for a survey that was sent to a wider sample of past and potential customers. The eight demanded qualities were:

1. More comprehensive evaluations

2. More comprehensive reports

3. Definition of all findings as pre- or postinjury

4. Better work capacity assessments

5. More treating physician follow-through with recommendations

6. More acceptance of findings at appeal hearings

7. Maintenance of independence from insurers

8. More understandable reports

The survey asked customers to rank each of these qualities using a five-point scale. Again using a five-point scale, respondents were also asked to rank their perception of how well the team's organization satisfied these qualities and their perception of the performance of three competitors using the same scale. The results of the survey were used to select targets for customer satisfaction that would distinguish the organization from the competition for the important demanded qualities.

The voice of the customer was translated into the organization's language by identifying what should be measured (performance measure) to predict customer satisfaction. The relative importance of performance measures is influenced by how many demanded qualities they predict and how effectively the demanded qualities are predicted. In this study, the six most important performance measures were:

1. The percent of symptoms identified

2. The percent of findings linked to observable data

3. The percent of findings separated into industrial or nonindustrial causes

4. The percent of job requirements simulated and tested

5. The percent of workers' treating physicians included in the process

6. The number of unexplained inconsistencies between observers

Targets for performance and units of measure were identified for each of the performance measures. The team then identified eleven functions that would need to be carried out to produce the demanded quality or to reach a target's performance measures:

1. Schedule evaluations prior to workers' arrival.

2. Survey workers prior to arrival.

3. Survey treating physicians prior to arrival.

4. Draft a summary of initial opinions by the end of day one.

5. Do custom work evaluations.

6. Do multiple trials of key functional tests.

7. Use quantitative measures for work evaluations.

8. Link all opinions to evidence.

9. Create one summary report.

10. Collect customer-satisfaction data at one month.

11. Collect outcome data at three months and one year.

The team took information gathered from customers about past failures in the service and, using tools of root cause analysis, identified two failure modes that strongly affect the service when not addressed:

1. Incomplete evaluations, noncompletion of requested activities by workers

2. Inconsistency in findings between different physician evaluators

After developing a high-level flowchart of the process, the team identified a series of critical tasks—the who, what, when, where, how, how much, and why of the task. The necessary training of the service team was carried out, and the new process was implemented. Customers reported glowing satisfaction with the changes in the service, and the rate of referrals for the service doubled.

To review, the QFD team identified targets, defined key actions necessary to reach these targets, and selected measures for assessing performance and feedback for navigating toward these targets. QFD, by design:

- Gets outside the boundaries of the organization and captures and ranks information from the environment

- Translates this information into organizational measures and targets

- Organizes the activity of people around these targets and measures to produce specific services that generate customer value

CASE OVERVIEW: THE TOOLS (500-FOOT VIEW)

The variation of QFD used for this study was presented in Figure 1.6:

Step 1	Capturing the voice of the customer
Step 2	Quality deployment
Step 3	Function deployment
Step 4	Failure mode deployment
Step 5	New process deployment
Step 6	Task Deployment

Step 1: Capturing the Voice of the Customer

Step 1 identifies key customer segments and generates a clearer understanding of customer concerns and needs by identifying demanded qualities. This step also ranks demanded qualities in order of their importance to the customer. Finally, this step produces a customer-generated analysis of the competition that ranks the QFD organization's performance in delivering these demanded qualities with the other choices available in the marketplace.

Three major customer segments were identified for this project:

1. The payer or insurer

2. The injured person

3. The injured worker's employer

For the sake of simplification and clarity, we focus only on the demanded qualities of the payer/insurer.

A nine-person project team was formed, including two nurses, two physicians, an occupational therapist, a physical therapist, and three representatives from sales and marketing. Members of this QFD team went into the field and interviewed claims managers, case managers, and legal personnel to gather data about what the customers wanted.

Members of the team went into the field to interview a small sample of customers, asking why and how the customers used the health-group services. The teams also constructed a high-level map of the customers' processes. Observations and the customers' spoken requirements were entered into a voice-of-the-customer table, Part 1 (VOCT1), which used the *who, what, when, where, why, and how format* as modified by Mazur (1996) (Figure 4.1). The goal was to capture the exact words of the customer. After each interview, the interview teams speculated about additional items or qualities that might enhance services. These items were also entered into the table. It was important at this point not to translate the language of the customer (*their* demanded quality) into technical language and professional jargon and idioms. To do so would most likely produce a map that recreated the provider's past instead of showing how to move into the future. The goal here is to discover what may already be there but is hidden by current biases.

Eighty unique items or requests were identified and entered into a VOCT1. Most QFD literature recommends a minimum of 15 or 20 individual customer interviews. In this project, the team interviewed 30 people "in the field," some in small groups of two to four and some individually.

After each interview, the customer's "voice" was expanded and separated as either demanded quality, performance measure, function, reliability item, failure mode, or other. This information was entered into the voice-of-the-customer table, Part 2 (VOCT2) (Figure 4.2):

- *Demanded qualities* are found by asking *why?* the customer uses the service. They are entered as positive statements for easier analysis later.

- *Performance measures* are a measurable technical assessment of a demanded quality. They state what is to be measured. In the QFD literature, performance measures are also called quality characteristics, quality attributes, or substitute quality characteristics.

- *Functions* are what the service does.

- *Reliability* describes the useful service time.

- *Failure modes* are the breakdown points in the service.

Of the 80 items identified, 61 were classified as demanded qualities. From the 30 people initially interviewed, a subgroup of 10 was assembled. The 61 demanded qualities were grouped and ranked in a hierarchy of importance by this subgroup using the affinity method, tree diagrams (Nayatani et al. 1988), and the analytical hierarchy process (AHP) (Saaty 1993). The affinity method was used to find natural groupings and the AHP was used to rank the groups and elements contained in each group. These tools are presented in more detail in Part 2. These interviews and the ranking took three full workdays, spread over a two-week period.

The data captured in the field was used to design a questionnaire that asked customers to use a five-point scale (1 for "does not matter" to 5 for "very strongly matters") to rank the eight demanded qualities identified as most important. The customers were also asked to rank the organization's services for these eight demanded qualities and those of competitors on a five-point scale (1 for "poor" to 5 for "excellent"). The survey was used to translate the qualitative data captured in the field into more quantitative data from a larger sample of the population of customers. The first two questions and the format of the questionnaire are shown in Figure 4.3, Part 1 and Part 2.

The same eight demanded qualities were entered into the rows of the quality-planning table. The overall format and the flow of information in the quality-planning

Cust Info	Voice of the Customer	Who, What, When, Where	Why	How	Reworded Data
	We want to know if drugs are involved.	Who: Nurse Case Manager What: Street Drugs When: Inpatient Evaluations Where: In Injured Worker	Find Illicit Drugs	Blood and Urine	We need screening for drugs.
	Except for name at the top, all the reports from some evaluation centers look and say the same thing.	Who: Legal Advocate What: Final Reports When: At Appeals Where: At Appeals	Credibility at Appeals	Individualized and Specific Case Reports	Individualized case-specific reports are created.
	Medical facts speak louder than medical opinions.	Who: Claims Examiner What: Distinguishing Criteria When: When Findings Contested Where: Negotiations or Appeals	Weight When Conflicting Opinions	Opinions Grounded by facts and Observations	Opinions are linked to facts wherever possible.
	Psychiatric impairments are barriers to vocational rehab.	Who: Nurse Case Manager What: Psychiatric Problems When: Getting Back to Work Where: In Vocational Retraining	Are Barriers to Return to Work	Motivation Reduced by Anxiety and Depression	Psychiatric issues can be barriers to return to work.
	Psychiatric problems are covered only if there was extreme danger at time of injury (i.e., victim of crimes).	Who: RN What: Psychiatric Problems When: Recommendations Where: Treatment	Reduce Frivolous Stress Claims	By Regulation	Only rarely is psychiatric treatment a covered benefit.

Figure 4.1. Sample voice-of-the-customer table, Part 1 (VOCT 1). The voice of the customer is captured by interviewing customers in the field, and the data is entered into the table.

Cust ID	Demanded Quality	Performance Measures	Function	Reliability	Failure Modes	Other
RN		Reports of Drug Screen				
Legal	Individualized and Case-Specific Reports					
CE		Opinion Linked to Facts				
CE				Identify psychiatric problems that could be barriers to retraining and work.		
RN					Recommend psychiatric or psychological treatments for noncovered conditions.	

Figure 4.2. Sample voice-of-the-customer table, Part 2 (VOCT 2). Data from the VOCT 1 is separated into demanded qualities, performance measures, functions, reliability, and failure mode.

51

Part 1. Using a scale where *1 = Does Not Matter* and *5 = Very Strongly Matters,* please rate how the following factors influence your decisions when deciding on whom to make a referral to for complex independent evaluations for injured workers.

	Does Not Matter	Somewhat Matters	Matters	Strongly Matters	Very Strongly Matters
1. Previous experience with the comprehensiveness of diagnostic medical evaluations	1	2	3	4	5
2. Previous experience with comprehensiveness of final reports	1	2	3	4	5

Part 2. Based on your experiences, please use the following scale to rate the providers on the items listed.

Scale

> 1 = *Poor*
> 2 = *Below Average*
> 3 = *Average*
> 4 = *Above Average*
> 5 = *Excellent*
> N = *No Experience*

	Rehabilitation Hospital	Competitor 1	Competitor 2
1. Comprehensiveness of the diagnostic medical evaluations	1 2 3 4 5 N	1 2 3 4 5 N	1 2 3 4 5 N
2. Comprehensiveness of the final reports	1 2 3 4 5 N	1 2 3 4 5 N	1 2 3 4 5 N

Figure 4.3. A questionnaire. Demanded qualities are used to construct a questionnaire to survey a larger population. Part 1 of the questionnaire asks customers to rank demanded qualities in order of importance. Part 2 of the questionnaire asks customers to rank how your organization performs relative to your competitors

table are shown in Figure 4.4. The columns on the left side of the table list data captured from customers:

- *Demanded qualities (DQs)*

- *Importance ratings,* a rating of the DQs' importance from the customers' perspective (survey data, Figure 4.3)

- *Customer competitive rankings,* a ranking of the provider and the competition from the customers' perspective (survey data, Figure 4.3)

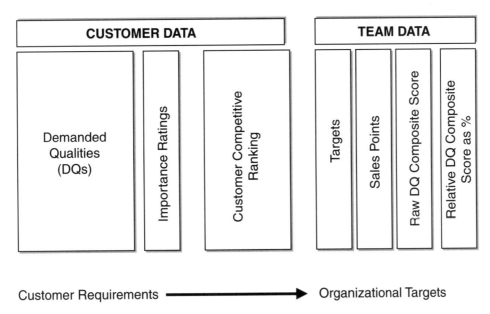

Customer Requirements ➔ Organizational Targets

Figure 4.4. Quality-Planning Table: general. The columns on the left-hand side of the Quality-Planning Table list data captured from customers as demanded qualities, the importance ratings of these demands from the customer's perspective, and the customer's competitive ranking of providers. Targets for improvement and sales points are derived from data and are listed on the right-hand side of the table along with composite scores.

Source: Journal on Quality Improvement (Oakbrook, Ill.: Joint Commission on Accreditation of Health-care Organizations, 1999), 300–315. Reprinted with permission.

The columns on the right side of the table are organizational assessments and objectives derived from the customer data:

- *Targets for improvement,* opportunities for organization improvement found by comparing the customers' perceived satisfaction from different sources and the importance ranking (Items that the customer ranked as important and for which the organization ranked low in comparison to the competition are opportunities for improvement.)

- *Sales points,* demanded qualities that would allow the service to distinguish itself from the competition or could be used to promote the service (These demanded qualities enhance the importance of the organization in the eyes of the customer.)

- *Composite scores,* the product of the importance rankings, targets for improvement, and sales points (Raw and relative demanded quality composite scores for each demanded quality are determined.)

Importance rank × Target ratio improvement × Sales point
= Raw DQ composite score

The quality-planning table for the case study is shown in Figure 4.5. Demanded qualities were entered into the rows of the first column of the table (column A). Customer importance rating and the competitive ranking from the survey were entered in the next two columns (Columns B and C, respectively).

The median customer importance ratings were either 5 (very strongly matters) or 4 (strongly matters) for all eight demanded qualities. There was no perceived difference by customers in the competitive rankings between potential suppliers for the first five demanded qualities listed on the table (rows 1 through 5). Though not dramatic, there were some perceived differences in the quality of the services for the last three items. The results of the survey confirmed that the demanded qualities identified by qualitative methods in the field were indeed quantitatively important. The competitive rankings also reinforced the organization's assessment that work was needed to improve and differentiate the perception of the organization's services.

To complete this table, the team:

1. Set a target for improvement (Column D, for each demanded quality Figure 4.5)

2. Calculated a ratio of improvement (Column E) by dividing the target for improvement by the current customer's ranking

3. Determined sales points (Column F) as 1.5, 1.2, or 1.0

4. Weighted the relative importance of each demanded quality (Column G), by multiplying the rating from the customer survey (Column B) by the magnitude of planned improvement (Column E, and the rank of each sales point (Column F) to yield the Raw demanded quality composite score.

5. Expressed each row's raw composite demanded quality score as a percent of the total weight of the eight demanded qualities for ease of comparison and communication (column H)

The demanded qualities captured in the field as the voice of the customer are "weighted" by organizational assessments of what is possible (target of improvement) and marketable (sales points). The results are used as input for the next step.

Step 1 answered the questions:

- What do customers want and need?

- Which of their wants and needs do they perceive as most important?

- How are we currently perceived in generating these demanded qualities when compared with available alternatives?

- What is the weighted importance to us for improving these demanded qualities?

Defining demanded qualities generates targets for the service. Like the messenger RNA in the cell, these targets set direction and shape the space where future actions will unfold. Like templates, these targets call forth sets of coordinated actions that unfold within the organization. In chapter 6, a number of tools and strategies are discussed to identify what may be missing and what may be hidden by our preexisting biases.

Demanded Qualities	Customer Survey Importance Rating	Our Organization	Competitor 1	Competitor 2	Competitor 3	Target	Ratio of Improvement	Sales Points	DQ Composite Importance	% Composite Importance
	B	C	C	C	C	D	E	F	G	H
1. More Comprehensive Evaluations	5	4	4	4	4	4	1	1.5	7.5	14.6
2. More Comprehensive Reports	5	4	4	4	4	5	1.25	1.5	9.38	18.2
3. Define All Findings as Press or Postinjury	5	4	4	4	4	5	1.25	1.5	9.38	18.2
4. Better Work Capacity Assessments	4	4	4	4	4	5	1.25	1.2	6.0	11.7
5. More MD Follow-Through with Recommendations	4	3	3	3	3	4	1.3	1.2	6.4	12.4
6. More Acceptance of Findings at Hearings	4	4	3	3	4	4	1	1.2	4.8	9.3
7. Independen ce From Insurers	4	4	3	4	4	4	1	1.0	4.0	7.8
8. More Understandable Reports	4	4	3	4	4	4	1	1.0	4.0	7.8

Figure 4.5. Quality-planning table: actual data. The table lists demanded qualities customer importance ratings captured from the survey (Column B) and competitive comparison of delivery of these services (Columns C) captured by the surveys. Targets for improvement (Column D), ratio of improvement (Column E) and sales point rankings (Column F) are identified. A raw composite importance score (Column G) and a weighted (percent) composite importance (Column H) are calculated. The composite importance is also shown graphically.

55

Step 2: Quality Deployment

This step translates the voice of the customer into the voice of the design team and, eventually, the voice of the organization. This is accomplished by a relationship matrix that includes the following elements (Figure 4.6):

- *Demanded qualities (rows)* identified in Step 1 are entered into the rows of the matrix along with their relative importance ratings.

- *Performance measures (columns)* are identified for each demanded quality as a way to assess and predict customer satisfaction.

- *Strength of relationships (each cell),* the predictive ability of a performance measure, is evaluated for each demanded quality.

- *Weight of each cell (for cells)* is determined by multiplying the cell by the relative importance rating for the corresponding demanded quality.

- A *weighted scores (for columns)* for a performance measure is the sum of the values in the column. The result is converted into a relative score as a percent.

The weighted scores plus other considerations for the performance measures are used to decide which measures are carried to Step 3. When completed, this relationship matrix plus the quality-planning table are called the *house of quality,* which translates the voice of the customer into organizational measures.

The Demanded Qualities/Performance Measures Matrix for the case study is shown in Figure 4.7. The data from the quality-planning table from Step 1 becomes the input for the rows of the Demanded Qualities/Performance Measures Matrix (labeled A). The relative composite score for each row is entered into the first column (labeled B). Free-association techniques, such as brainstorming, were used to generate lists of performance measures for each demanded quality. These were entered into the columns of the matrix (labeled C). Then, working cell by cell, the team assessed the relationship between each performance measure (column) and demanded quality (row). The question was asked, "If you knew the results of the performance measure (column), how predictive would it be for the demanded quality (row)?" The team used ● to symbolize a strong relationship, ◑ for a medium relationship, and ○ for a weak relationship. The cell was left blank if no relationship existed. Next, the weighted importance for each performance measure was calculated by multiplying the strength of the correlation in each cell (9, 3, 1, 0) in the column by the relative composite score of the row, summing the columns, and expressing the sum of each column as a percent of the total of all the columns (labeled D). These calculations identify the columns that most highly correlate with all the rows. This matrix analysis selects those performance measures that are most important for satisfying the customer (labeled E). Target values are selected that best satisfy the customer within the goals and objectives of the organization (labeled F). The five most highly weighted performance measures and the performance measure percent workers' treating physicians included in process were selected by the team for driving the project.[1]

---

[1]The rationale for carrying *percent workers' treating physicians included in the process* forward even though its weight was less than half the next lowest selected measure (4.7 versus 12.1), and for not including row 2 from quality-planning table (*More comprehensive reports*) forward is discussed in Part 2.

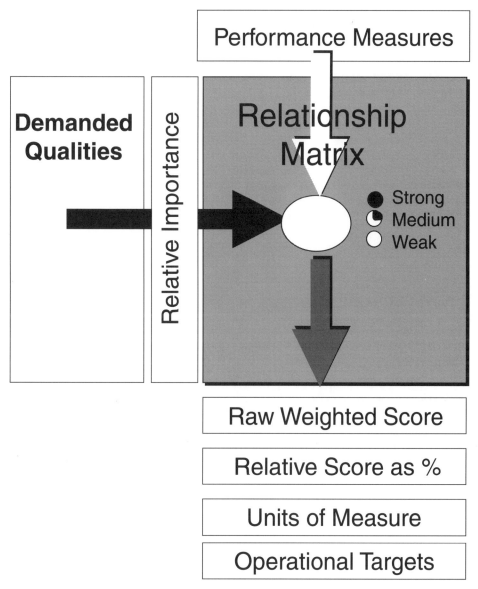

Figure 4.6. Matrix tool: general. The relationship matrix translates the voice of the customer into the voice of the organization. Demanded qualities, rows, are translated into performance measures (the hows of measurements). The strength of the column in predicting the demanded quality of each row is estimated as strong, medium, weak, or blank. The performance measures in the columns with strongest correlations are carried to the next matrix.

Source: Journal on Quality Improvement (Oakbrook, Ill.: Joint Commission on Accreditation of Healthcare Organizations, 1999), 300–315. Reprinted with permission.

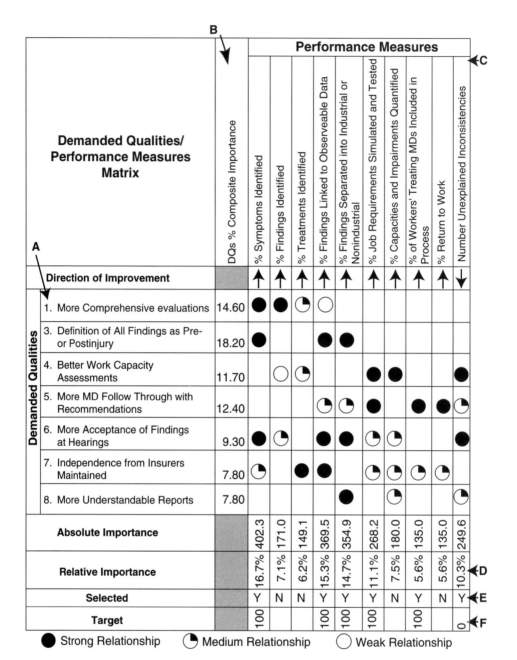

Figure 4.7. Demanded Quality/Performance Measures Matrix. This matrix is often referred to as the *House of Quality*. It compares the relationship between demanded qualities (A) and performance measures (C, measurable quality characteristics) for these. Cell by cell, the strength of each performance measure's (columns) ability to predict each demanded quality (rows) is rated as ● strong, ◐ medium, ○ weak, or blank. The strength of the relationships within the cell is then weighted by multiplying it by the importance rating (B) of the demanded quality. Those columns that are strongly correlated with demanded qualities are selected to be carried to the next matrix (E). Specific units of measures for each performance measure and targets are identified for these measures (F).

Source: Figures and calculations for matrices done with software from QualiSoft, 4652 Patrick Rd., West Bloomfield, Mich. 48233, qualisoft@aol.com. (We have no financial relationship with QualiSoft.) Demo available www.qualisoft.com.

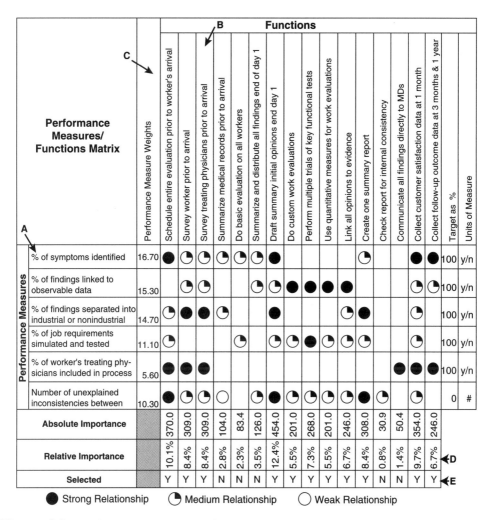

Figure 4.8. Performance Measures/Functions Matrix. This matrix translates performance measures into functions necessary to satisfy the customer requirements. The importance of performance measures is used to identify important functions.

Step 2 answered the questions:

- What quantitative performance measures will be used to evaluate actions required to ensure that demanded qualities were delivered?
- How important are these performance measures?
- What are our desired operational targets for each measure?

Step 3: Function Deployment

Step 3 identifies the organizational functions that have the greatest impact on the performance measures selected in Step 2. The six performance measures identified in Step 2 became the input to the rows of a Performance Measures/Functions Matrix (labeled A, Figure 4.8).

Key functions for meeting demanded qualities or performance measures are identified and entered into the columns (labeled B). Cell by cell, the strength of the relationship between each row and column was determined as strong, medium, or weak by asking the question, "How important is this function in producing the target for the performance measure?" The cells and columns were weighted by matrix calculations similar to those described for Step 2, except that here the columns were multiplied by the performance measures weight for each row (labeled C). The columns were summed, and the importance of each column was identified as a percent of the total sum of columns (labeled D). Eleven key functions were identified to be carried through the next step (labeled E).

Not every conceivable function is carried forward, only key functions critical to the process. Models of chaotic systems indicate that not every step within the system needs to be regulated or controlled to stabilize the system (Pribram 1991; Kauffman 1993). Rather, if reinforcing and balancing feedback is built into a few key steps as these steps become ordered, the rest of the system resonates with them and organizes itself around this stabilizing center. Similarly, the goal in QFD is first to identify key functions and critical tasks and then to identify measurable characteristics for feedback. This feedback is then used to consistently produce services that the customer will recognize as satisfying or exceeding his or her expectations.

Step 3 answered the question:

- What key functions are needed to influence the performance measures?

Step 4: Failure Mode Deployment

Step 4 is designed to identify how a process is likely to fail. The functions identified in Step 3 were entered into a Functions/Failure Mode Matrix (Figure 4.9). Data from the failure mode column of the VOCT, as well as complaints, incident report data, and past experience of the team regarding where the process tended to unravel, were all reviewed. The potential failure modes were entered into the columns, and the cells and columns were weighted and compared using matrix calculations similar to those in Steps 2 and 3. The two items *incomplete evaluations, noncompletion of requested activities by workers* and *inconsistency in findings between different physician evaluators* were identified as the most highly weighted potential failure modes and selected to be addressed.

Step 4 answered the question:

- How are the functions likely to fail?

Step 5: New Process Deployment

The QFD team assessed the current process as inadequate to perform some key functions. Parts of the process had to be redesigned. Lists of alternative concepts that might perform the needed functions were generated. Concepts for strengthening the functions around potential breakdown points identified in Step 4 were also evaluated.

The team identified *create one summary report* as a key function in the Performance Measures/Function Matrix (Figure 4.9) and *inconsistencies in findings between different physician evaluators* as a highly weighted potential failure mode. Three alternative

Functions/Failure Mode Matrix	Weight of Functions	Incomplete evaluations, workers not completing requested activities	Having to add additional procedures and tests during evaluation period	Failure of team to adapt to unforeseen circumstances	Breakdown in team following policies and procedures	After evaluation period, discover some critical tasks are incomplete	Inconsistent findings between different physician evaluators
Schedule entire evaluation prior to workers' arrival.	10.1	●	◗		●		
Survey workers prior to arrival.	8.40	●		◗	◗		◗
Survey treating physician prior to arrival.	8.40		●	◗	◗		◗
Draft summary of initial opinions by the end of day one.	12.4		●	◗		◗	●
Do custom work evaluations.	5.50	●				◗	○
Perform multiple trials of key functional tests.	7.30					◗	○
Use quantitative measures for work evaluations.	5.50				◗	◗	
Link all opinions to evidence.	6.70					◗	◗
Create one summary report.	8.40		○				●
Collect customer-satisfaction data at one month.	9.70	●				●	●
Collect follow-up outcome data at three months and one year.	6.70					◗	
Absolute Importance		303	225	87.6	157	219	357
Relative Importance		22.4%	16.7%	6.5%	11.7%	16.2%	26.5%
Selected		Y	N	N	N	N	Y

● Strong Relationship   ◗ Medium Relationship   ○ Weak Relationship

Figure 4.9. Functions/Failure Mode Matrix. This matrix is used to identify and rank failure modes for functions.

design concepts to accomplish this were identified (columns in Figure 4.10). One concept involved a series of phone calls; another involved a series of faxes; and the third involved a face-to-face meeting of all consulting physicians.

These functions were competitively ranked (King 1989) based on organizational time required, cycle or turnaround time, cost, and consistency. Based on this ranking, Concept 2 was selected as the best. Concept 2 is one potential solution to failure mode *inconsistency in findings between different physician evaluators.*

Each of the concepts in Figure 4.10 contained a feedback loop. A key strategy to deploying reliable and robust systems is to included self-regulating feedback at steps critical to the process. For example, the same customers with this concern had previously complained about long delays in getting reports. The root cause of this failure was identified as delays in the consulting physicians getting their reports back to the organization.

Once the breakdown was identified, a definite time commitment for completion of the report by each physician expert was agreed to: one week after completion of their evaluation. A new step to check that these conditions of satisfaction were met was added, and, if conditions were not met, immediate and balancing feedback to the provider (physician) was generated by a phone call. As shown in Figure 4.11, redesigning the process at this step resulted in a reduction of total cycle time (from when the injured worker was discharged until the final report was in the hands of the insurer) from a mean of 50 days to 18 days (Chaplin 1996). The same strategy was used to generate one common report by physicians for this current project.

Step 5 answered the questions:

- What is the best overall design to deliver key functions for the best service?

- Where is reinforcing and balancing feedback needed to shape and inform team behavior?

Step 6: Task Deployment

Identified from flowcharts and placed in a task-deployment table, key tasks, equipment, facilities, tools, and training are the "hows" that are needed to achieve the best concept. The who, what, where, and so on were then identified and communicated to the people who would be accountable for these tasks, equipment, facilities, tools, training, and so on (Figure 4.12).

By the time the project team reached task deployment, functions and tasks that had been identified earlier for facilitating and improving the efficiency of key steps in the evaluation process had already been incorporated into day-to-day practices by those members of the QFD team who also participated in the evaluation of injured workers. This occurred prior to the formal deployment of specific tasks. That is, the ongoing process of providing this service had already evolved and incorporated some strategies that made the staff's day-to-day work activity easier and more efficient. In contrast, those tasks that required new sets of actions that were primarily to measure performance and functions—such as follow-up satisfaction surveys and checks for internal consistency—required more effort to incorporate and accomplish in a consistent manner.

Step 6 answered the question:

- Who will do what, where, when, why, and how; and how much will it cost?

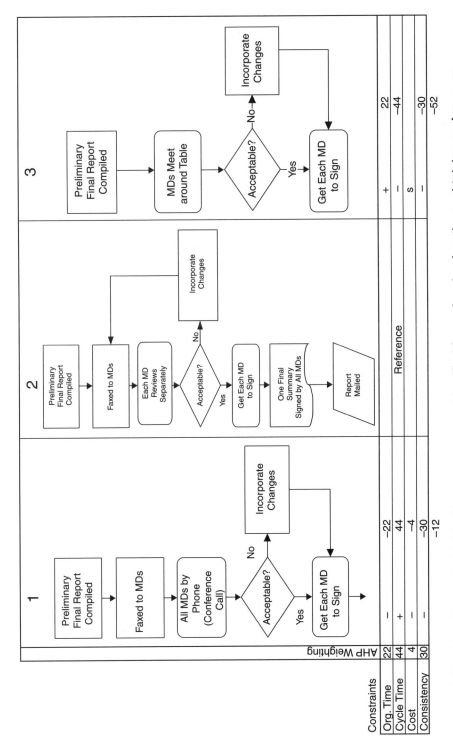

Figure 4.10. New Concepts Matrix. New concepts are identified for performing functions, obtaining performance measures, or delivering demanded qualities. Competing functions are ranked based on weighted criteria, and the most heavily weighted concepts are selected.

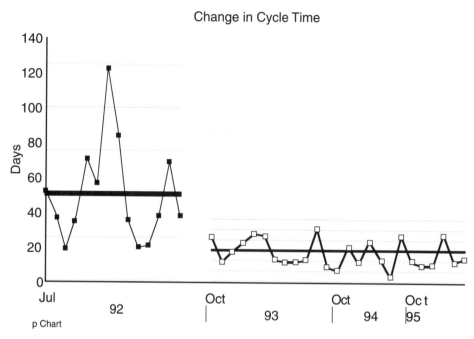

Figure 4.11. Comprehensive evaluation process: feedback to improve quality and reduce variation. When the feedback loop was added to reinforce our target, the cycle time from the time of patient arrival to the time of delivering a comprehensive final report decreased from an average of 50 days to 18 days. As shown in the control chart, the variation in the output was also dramatically reduced.

Source: Ed Chaplin, "Re-engineering in Healthcare: Chain Hand Off and the Four-Phase Work Cycle," *Quality Progress* 29 (October 1996). Reprinted with permission.

PRELIMINARY OUTCOMES

A five-year experience with this same customer base showed an average of 22 (±4) evaluations per year (Figure 4.13). The QFD project started with interviews in the field during August of 1997, and the new system was implemented in November of 1997. Formal and informal feedback from customers after implementation was extremely positive. During 1998, the number of referrals for the service doubled.

As we discuss in Part 2, it is not always necessary to go through all these steps for every project. Sometimes key data from early steps is incorporated into existing process. For example, specific measures identified in a Demanded Quality/Performance Measures matrix (also called the *house of quality*) can be directly and successfully incorporated into current tasks and functions.

COMMENTS

People within most healthcare organizations believe they are sincere and capable when they state that they want to respond to their customers with improved services, whether the *customer* is the patient, family, physician, insurer, or community. The healthcare

What	Who	When	Where	How	How Much	Why	Other
All planning and preadmit scheduling is complete.	Marketing Secretary	Start 3 weeks prior to planned admit.	CRHSD	Phone and Fax		Build template for evaluation.	
Send and collect preadmit scheduling patient questionnaire	Marketing Secretary	Send 2 weeks before planned admit.	CRHSD	Mail Phone		Build complete list of symptoms and impairments.	
Send and make call questionnaire to treating physician.	Marketing Secretary Managing MD Peer to Peer	Survey 2 weeks. Call 1 week.	CRHSD	Mail Phone		Build complete list of symptoms, diagnoses, and impairments.	

Figure 4.12. Task-Deployment Table. The task-deployment table identifies critical tasks. The who, what, when, where, why, and how of the task are determined along with any tools and training that may be needed.

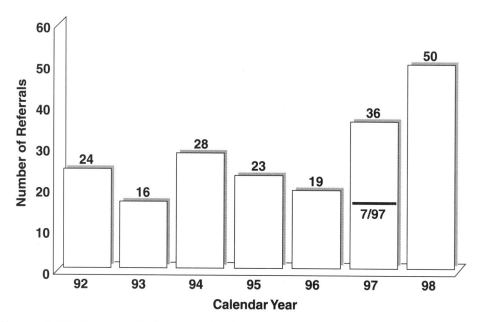

Figure 4.13. Some preliminary results. The redesign project started in August of 1997 and was implemented in November of 1997. In 1998, the rate of new referrals slightly more than doubled.

worker's desire, however, does not consistently show up in services. This is in part due to a blindness to cultural presuppositions and historical barriers that constrain innovation and change. These presuppositions and barriers keep us focused on our *as is* maps of the world.

Some ineffectiveness can also be attributable to trying to respond to too many and too divergent a stream of unsystematic feedback and demands. When trying to incorporate too many new targets, teams become overwhelmed by the complexity and revert to the perceived safety of their old ways. At other times, a great deal of work goes into incorporating a voiced need that is peculiar to one or two customers but is not highly valued by most customers. Another barrier to incorporating improvements in healthcare services is that important needs brought back by someone in sales or marketing are often discounted and dismissed by the healthcare professionals delivering the service.

When important demanded qualities are identified and the journey of change begins, the team may fail to anticipate failure modes or to design a reinforcing and balancing feedback process coupled with rewards and consequences. This is a necessary element in changing human behavior.

Sometimes there are experiences of selecting appropriate targets, designed processes, but failing to introduce the necessary tools and training to staff. The effort fails. It is ironic that one of the core competencies of rehabilitation hospitals is to help patients overcome their impairments by reinforced and repetitive practice, yet these same organizations repeatedly expect to change staff behavior by memos and didactic classroom presentations.

Many healthcare organizations have achieved some successes but not consistently enough to substantially change the organization and to overcome the culture of paternalism and denial that is so deeply ingrained in healthcare that it is usually transparent to healthcare workers. QFD is a set of tools and practices that can assist our industry in overcoming some of these obstacles and consistently enhance and improve our services. We talk about being patient/customer focused, but, for the most part, healthcare is still provider focused. The things that get done are those that are easy or routine from the provider's perspective. If we want to change this pattern, we need to identify what is important to patients, then intervene and modify our actions at a level that changes what is habitual or routine. QFD can be used to shift organizational awareness from self-centered, provider-focused maps shaped by our hidden presuppositions to sensory-based, customer-focused maps that assist in defining and delivering what is important to the customers.

Throughout the QFD process, there is a dynamic tension between creating a definition for the process as a whole and jumping to the details of the parts (that is, specific tasks and roles). We are conditioned to jump toward immediate action—the task at hand. A challenge in the early practice of QFD is staying focused on the larger context of the whole, the process, the organization, and the customer. The goal is to expand awareness of existing conditions before acting to deploy specific tasks and roles (the who will do what, etc.). Designing a broad outline of the whole entity—a vision with structure, sets of relationships, specific measures, and feedback and input from the environment—provides the context that informs and organizes the parts and establishes a balance between differentiation and integration. The risk of jumping to specific actions and roles too soon is that the final process will be fragmented or dominated by the needs of current roles in the organization and not the needs of the customer.

Our social organizations, as an extension of our biology, are structures with directions and boundaries for action, sets of interrelationships, internal flows of energy, and flows of signals from the environment. At any given moment, an organization functions only within the limits of the pattern of the system it has evolved to. When we say the system is broken or in error, we are making a claim relative to some expectation we have and not necessarily to something inherent in the system. No matter how much we complain about current situations, on close examination we usually find we are functioning in perfect alignment with the underlying historical pattern that is present and the reinforcing and balancing feedback that produces the stable whole we have become. The organization that continued to refer patients to physicians that they assessed as late in getting in their reports acted in a way that reinforced the current homeostatic relationships. For organizations to change functions, they must also change structures. However, building a future based on an uncertain and untested model requires giving up the perceived comforts and certainty of the past before the rewards of the uncertain future can be attained. Change involves risk, and risk provokes moods and emotions that inhibit change.

We would not expect a pancreatic islet cell, which has differentiated to generate and secrete insulin, to suddenly start producing digestive enzymes (though it retains the capacity to do so). This could not happen without first changing the cell's organizational structure—creating new RNA (targets), new protein enzymes (capacities for action), new feedback loops, and so on. This is equally true for our social organizations. Organizational functions match underlying structure. Attempts to substantially alter function without also altering structure are usually short-lived and ineffective. Like the lactic acid in the sprinter, by-products eventually accumulate and homeostatic mechanisms drive function back toward the underlying design that is already in place—the structure (anatomy), internal patterns and relationships (physiology), networks for the generation and exchange of value (biochemistry), and relationships with the environment (ecology).

The example presented here had a goal of improving a current process to attain a future still based primarily on the past competencies, an existing service. QFD can also be used to design and deploy future-based development (innovation). The innovative process can be triggered by identifying an unmet concern in the environment and determining what assessments would need to be produced to satisfy that concern. What are the demanded qualities? How will we measure if these qualities are being produced and delivered (attributes)? What competencies and functions will be required? And so on.

Patterns or strategies we can follow in our attempts to change our organizations (Spinosa, Flores and Dreyfus 1997) to meet the three challenges presented in chapter 3 include:

- Reconfiguring services around innovations

- Cross-appropriating knowledge and practices from other industries into our organizations

- Realigning our organizations around fundamental concerns for which we have lost our focus

In general, healthcare as a service industry lags behind other service industries in the area of quality management. The strategies and practices of QFD can be cross-appropriated into healthcare. To survive, healthcare organizations must be able to rapidly adapt to changing customer needs, differentiate new services, integrate these new services with old services, and align the organization around comparison purposes. Such organizations will have a competence in:

- Identifying customer wants (Voice-of-the-customer quality-planning tables)

- Identifying gaps between wants and current provided services (quality-planning table)

- Identifying new targets (feed-forward measures; quality-planning table)

- Identifying a few specific measures that will be used to navigate and determine whether or not actions are moving toward the targets (performance measures)

- Identifying already inherent competencies and providing any missing tools and training necessary to produce these measures (failure mode deployment and task deployment)

- Coupling feedback measures with employee rewards and consequences to reinforce the learning of new practices (new concepts matrix and task deployment)

These are all key elements to successful renewal and change efforts, whether they involve innovation, cross-appropriation, rediscovery, or reconfiguration around core concerns and values. By designing and building environments that contain feed-forward and feedback measures coupled to organizational and individual rewards and consequences, QFD can be used to shift managerial emphasis from managing individual people to designing contexts where evolving and self-organizing services emerge.

Once the members of a QFD team have learned the process, completed a project, and articulated the process and the significance of their findings to their organization and peers, they will never see customers, providers, services, and their organization in the same way. Instead, their view of the organization and its many parts will be permanently changed, and their own ability to function effectively in the organization will expand.

Unless you already have some working knowledge of QFD, the material in this chapter may seem overwhelming. Keep in mind that our goal to this point has been to provide an appreciation for the structure (anatomy), sets of relationships (physiology), types of actions and feedback measures (biochemistry), and a methodology for capturing information that couples your organization to your environment (ecology). These tools, like enzymes, lower the energy necessary for change by identifying key roles, functions, structures, and systems to produce targeted results. The details are in Part I.

Part II

Step-by-Step
Healthcare QFD

Chapter 5
Organizational Readiness

Upon completing this chapter, you will be able to:

- Reflect on the organizational gap between the current structure and being customer driven.

- Plan your QFD project.

- Integrate QFD into your process to design or redesign a service or facility.

- Ask useful questions.

Human beings have bound together into social organizations to create units that have more value than they would as individuals. The generation and exchange of value with its environment, the community, are the sustaining life force of any social organization. QFD is a catalyst for generation and exchange.

Traditional marketing techniques such as focus groups, surveys, and customer-satisfaction reports are used to capture data from the environment, but these methods do not provide the same level of detail as a comprehensive QFD process. QFD embodies and integrates multiple practices and sets of tools to examine the customer needs in detail from a variety of perspectives. Some examples include *going to the Gemba,* the *Kano model,* and *up-front loading of resources.* To more fully understand customers, an organization must go to the customer's environment and actually observe the customer using the product or service. This provides members of the team with firsthand experience of how their products or services fit into the customer's work and world. It offers the team an opportunity to use all senses (sight, sound, touch, and sometimes smell and taste) in the customer's environment and an opportunity to reveal their individual and collective assumptions about what customers want. This gives a richer perspective than can be grasped from surveys or focus groups. The Japanese call this type of market research "going to the Gemba."

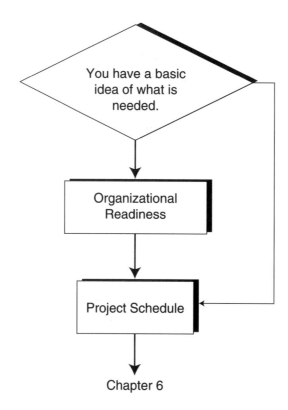

You have a basic idea of what is needed.

Organizational Readiness

Project Schedule

Chapter 6

Two *kanji* symbols form the Gemba character. The first is that of a king overlooking his domain. The second symbolizes the land and the swineherds laboring under the sun. Together they symbolize the importance of understanding the customer's environment and his or her behavior in that environment. How do you do that? By actually going to and talking to customers, observing their action (processes), and recording what they say. The most effective way of doing this is to actually work with the customers, that is, *be* the customer. Organizations such a AT&T Bell Laboratories have team members work in the customer's organization for two to three months as part of their QFD projects.

The *Kano model* is another important tool in the QFD process. Use of the Kano method with products has demonstrated that improvements in the performance of what is seen as a basic need does not produce a more satisfied customer; rather, it is the features of products or services that are unexpected or exciting that increase customer satisfaction.

QFD emphasizes up-front planning. Do it right the first time. Many service organizations anticipate allocating most of their deployment resources just before and after the time of start-up. They operate on the premise that planning before implementation will be inadequate and that expecting quality problems as the service begins to be delivered is unavoidable. Like the phenomenon of the Ames's room and the placebo, this perspective generates limiting targets that become self-fulfilling. We end up doing what we have always done to get things going and attempt to patch up deficiencies later.

The cell spends 90% to 95% of its response time after an environmental stimulus evaluating the stimulus within the context of its organization as a whole. Then, after determining what is important, the cell designs and deploys a target. Setting the best target for any improvement process is critical. The target calls forth the actions necessary to reach it. Fuzzy or sloppy targets yield fuzzy and sloppy results.

EXERCISE 5.1

- Break up into groups of three to six people.
- If this is an educational or training QFD project, brainstorm several possible healthcare services that you would find interesting. Select one to be used in the workshops throughout this book.
- If this is an application project, try a small project first, for example, a hospital cafeteria. Pick a project that is likely to be successful. The experience gained by doing the exercise will help you in larger, more complex applications.

EXERCISE 5.2

- Draw a high-level process map showing how your organization currently goes about improving or redesigning a process or service.
- Use symbols familiar to the team (those you usually use), or define a set of symbols.
- The flowchart should have no more than 20 steps in the process, preferably less.
- This is the *as is* process.
- If the team cannot agree on the *as is* process, what does this tell you?
- If the team does agree, what constraints do you see in the current process?

WHERE ARE WE NOW? A READINESS PICTURE

Before we go to the Gemba, we need to know where we are starting. We need to build the space within which the QFD project can emerge. We do this by identifying and constructing targets and feedback that integrate and self-organize the project space. In this section, you will complete a *radar chart* that illustrates organizational readiness. When your readiness has been determined, you will generate a project flowchart and a project schedule, a network of commitments.

A radar chart is a simple graphic method for assessing where your organization is with respect to the basic principles that support QFD. The radar chart shown in Figure 5.1 has five dimensions:

- We are customer driven.

- We know our customers.

- We invest resources up front to determine customer needs.

- All functions impacted by a service participate in designing it.

- We understand the context in which our services are sought.

A nine-point scale is used to record how well each statement describes your current organization. The *1* near the center of the circle (see figure) indicates that the statement describes the opposite of your organization. A *9* on the perimeter indicates that the statement describes your organization precisely. For example, consider the statement, "We are customer driven." If this truly describes your organization accurately, you would score a *9*. If you are still primarily provider focused, you would score a *1*.

Throughout Part 2 of the text, we will use the case example presented in chapter 4 to illustrate the steps and tools of the QFD process. The QFD team in our case study completed the radar chart in Figure 5.1. They assessed their organization as strong in

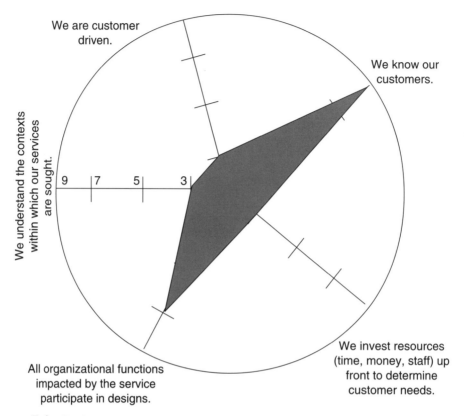

Figure 5.1. Radar chart: a readiness picture. This graphic is a self-assessment tool. Where is your organization with respect to the basic principles that support QFD in the five dimensions shown in the figure?

knowing who the primary customer was and fairly successful in getting cross-functional department participation in producing designs. They assessed themselves as weak in investing resources up front in order to produce a robust design, as well as in understanding the context in which their service was used by the customer and in truly being customer driven. These observations could be used to select the components of the QFD process that would provide the largest improvement.

Too many people are under the impression that every application of QFD must use the entire QFD process. This is not true. Use whatever components match your current need, willingness, resources, and time line. Comprehensive QFD involves a number of steps and tools. Not every QFD effort needs to use every tool. What is used depends on what data is already available, whether the project is to design a new service or redesign an existing service, and so on. Because this book introduces QFD and is designed to be used as a workbook, we present QFD in a comprehensive manner using all its tools. Comments are included to explain where different components are used. In presenting a comprehensive model of QFD for healthcare, we present the technically correct processes. However, the realities of actual projects may suggest process modifications. We will identify the modifications made by the team in the case study while doing their first QFD.

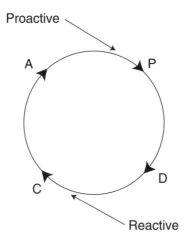

Figure 5.2. PDCA: Demming cycle. The *Plan, Do, Check, Act* cycle is as critical a process to the delivering of healthcare services as the scientific method is to the practice of medicine.

EXERCISE 5.3

Use the blank radar chart in Appendix A and record your perception of your organization. A common pitfall here is all or none thinking. If all scores are high, results might reflect a lack of awareness on the part of the team or a lack of honesty. Scores that are all *1*s might be more reflective of the team or organizational mood rather than the reality; most organizations that have been around awhile do something well.

CRITICAL PROCESSES

As noted in chapter 3, capturing stimuli from the environment, evaluating these stimuli, projecting targets for action, acting, and checking feedback from these actions are a critical process for the cell. This process is fundamental to life itself. It manifests itself in medicine as the scientific method:

- Create a hypothesis.
- Design an experiment to test the hypothesis.
- Collect data and compare the results of the experiment to the hypothesis.
- Accept, reject, or modify the hypothesis.

It manifests in the field of quality as in the *PDCA* or *Deming cycle* (Figure 5.2). The classic definition of PDCA is:

- *Plan*—Create a model to be tested.
- *Do*—Try the model.
- *Check*—Compare actual results and predicted results.
- *Act*—Modify or solidify the theory.

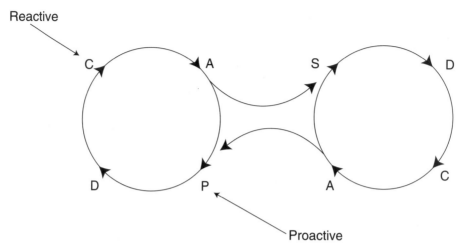

Figure 5.3. PCDA–SDCA cycle interactions. The *Standards, Do, Check, Act* cycle is a steady-state institutionalized version of the PDCA cycle. Standards rather than planned targets call forth the actions of the organization's processes.

As a result of CQI and TQM initiatives, most healthcare organizations are familiar with the PDCA cycle. The PDCA cycle is as critical a process to an organization as the scientific method is to medicine. The PDCA cycle can be and is often used retrospectively. It is deployed after a breakdown is identified. It can also be used proactively as a map for the design process or even to create an organizational structure. The PDCA cycle has no end point, but is instead a continuous improvement process. After several times around the PDCA cycle, an organization will be satisfied with the performance of the system. Once this level is reached, the cycle becomes institutionalized as the *SDCA cycle.* The *S* stands for *standardize.* In other words, the organization establishes one way to support its customers:

- *Standardize*—Establish a successful model.

- *Do*—Try the model.

- *Check*—Compare actual results and predicted results.

- *Act*—Modify or solidify the theory.

This cycle is used for monitoring the performance of the system. If performance becomes unsatisfactory, the process returns to the PDCA cycle (Figure 5.3).

In this text, we will use this PDCA schema as a tool to build both high-level and detailed maps for designing and redesigning projects. In QFD, we start the cycle with *C, checking* what customers in a particular market want. We follow a *CAPDCA variation* of the cycle:

- *Check* the current market.

- *Act* to improve current service.

- *Plan* new service.

- *Do* or implement the service.

- *Check* the performance.

- *Act* with corrective measures, if needed.

Each high-level step has a nested subordinate CAPDCA cycle to accomplish its task, as shown in Figure 5.4. The project flow map becomes a high-level template for a more detailed project schedule (Figure 5.4). For each phase of the project, a project schedule identifies a purpose or target, the task to be performed, and the promises of who will do what, how, and by when (conditions of satisfaction). The project schedule includes a document(s) to be used as a tool for each task. That document, when completed, is evidence that conditions of satisfaction have been met.

In our experience, many teams do not outline these steps in any great detail. They are discussed casually, glazed over, or skipped entirely. However, just as when you reach out and touch an object, it is the clarity of the target that calls forth the necessary actions. Setting out before the team and the organization a vividly clear target with measures and conditions of satisfaction for reaching that target is invaluable for calling forth and coordinating the necessary actions for the project to be successful.

Lacking a sense of how the project fits together as a whole, roles of the individual parts become blurred and conflicts arise between the parts. Experience also suggests that such detailed levels of commitment, that is, promises for future results in projects that are critical to patient care, often provoke anxiety in healthcare professions. Responses arise such as "patient care is too complex to be able to say we will have these problems resolved by such and such a time." When designing projects, particularly around failure points, healthcare professions are prone to chain every event to the worse outcome—death. This predisposition can have two consequences. First, uncertainty generated can paralyze a team. Second, casting the redesign process as both complex and dangerous blocks action, allowing things to stay as they are, that is, making the task sound impossible eliminates the risk of attempting to change. These tendencies provoke emotions that drive teams back from Point 2 to Point 1 of the map of change (see Figure 2.9).

EXERCISE 5.4

Create a project flowchart:
- Develop a high-level project flowchart following the example in Figure 5.4.
- What documents will be used as tools and evidence of satisfaction, that is, for completion of each step? If this is your first exposure to QFD and is a training exercise, leave the document columns blank for now and fill them in when these steps are covered in later exercises. This will allow you to develop a sense of how the parts fit together to form a whole.
- If this is an actual project, this and the following project schedule are critical to building a clear target and aligning organizational support for the project.

EXERCISE 5.5

Develop a project schedule:
- Develop a project schedule following the example in Figure 5.5.
- Again, if this is the first QFD project, fill in the document as described for Workshop 5.4 (Appendix A).

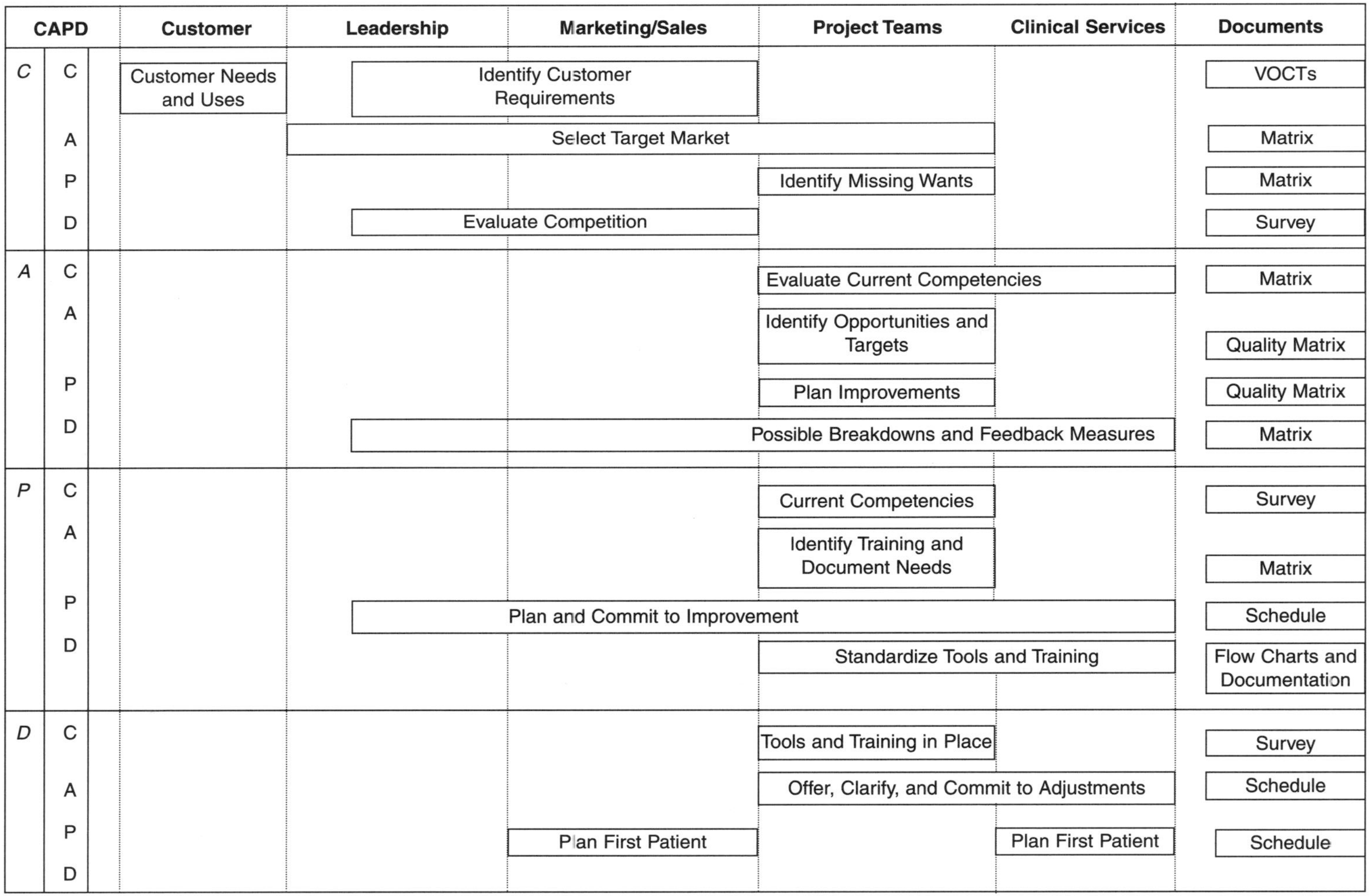

CAPD		Customer	Leadership	Marketing/Sales	Project Teams	Clinical Services	Documents
C	C	Customer Needs and Uses	Identify Customer Requirements				VOCTs
	A			Select Target Market			Matrix
	P				Identify Missing Wants		Matrix
	D			Evaluate Competition			Survey
A	C				Evaluate Current Competencies		Matrix
	A				Identify Opportunities and Targets		Quality Matrix
	P				Plan Improvements		Quality Matrix
	D				Possible Breakdowns and Feedback Measures		Matrix
P	C				Current Competencies		Survey
	A				Identify Training and Document Needs		Matrix
	P			Plan and Commit to Improvement			Schedule
	D				Standardize Tools and Training		Flow Charts and Documentation
D	C				Tools and Training in Place		Survey
	A				Offer, Clarify, and Commit to Adjustments		Schedule
	P			Plan First Patient			Schedule
	D					Plan First Patient	Schedule

Figure 5.4. Project flowchart. The project flowchart identifies functions that need to be carried out across different departments and the documents that will serve as evidence that these functions have been completed.

Project Schedule

Start date 7/16/97

PHASE	PURPOSE	TASKS	WHO	WHEN	HOW	DOCUMENT
Check Current Market	Capture data about current wants and opportunities for innovation.	C: Capture voice of the customer.	Marketing	8/15/97	Customer Visits	VOCT1
		A: Order data.	Marketing	8/15/97	Affinity, Tree, and AHP	Affinity, Tree, and AHP
		P: Identify and clarify key missing wants.	Marketing	8/15/97	Customer Survey	VOCT2
		D: Evaluate competition.	Marketing	9/12/97	Customer Survey	Horizontal of Matrix
Act to improve our current service	Identify and offer process improvements.	C: Evaluate current service.	Marketing	9/12/97	Customer Survey	Horizontal of Matrix
		A: Identify opportunities.	Project Team	10/12/97	Quality Planning Matrix	House of Quality
		P: Plan improvements.	Project Team	10/17/97	Relationship Matricies	House of Quality
		D: Feedback Mechanisms and Failure Analyses	Project Team	10/17/97	Brainstorming	Flowchart and Matrix
Plan Implementation	Commit to and deploy infrastructure.	C: Current Competencies	Project Team	10/17/97	Provider Survey	Matrix
		A: ID Training & Document Needs	Project Team	10/17/97	Forms and Competency Reviews	Checksheet
		P: Plan and commit to improvements.	Project Team	10/24/97	Schedule	Checksheet
		D: Standardize tools and training.	Project Team	11/1/97	Departmental Education	Tools/Training Checksheet
Do Implementation	Change service.	C: Tools and Processes in Place	Departments	10/27/97	Internal Survey	Checksheet
		A: Make any adjustments.	Departments	10/27/97	Departmental Education	Checksheet
		P: First Claim/Patient	Treatment Team	11/3/97	Implement Systems	Schedule
		D: Do	Treatment Team	11/1/97	Implement Systems	Patient Assessment
Check Outcomes	Assess customer satisfaction.	C: Assess customer satisfaction.	Marketing	Monthly	1 Wk, 3 Mo, 6 Mo F/U	Outcomes Table
		A: Offer adjustments.	Project Team	Monthly	Ad Hoc Project Team Meetings	Minutes
		P: Clarify and commit to adjustments.	Treatment Team	Monthly	Tools and Training	Minutes
		D: Deploy adjustments.	Treatment Team	Monthly		Checksheet

Figure 5.5. Project schedule. The project schedule identifies the tasks to be completed and also the who, the when, and the how these will be completed. The schedule also lists documents that will serve as evidence that the tasks are completed. The project schedule, when complete, is used as a target of the whole and a record of the commitments of the projects team.

SUGGESTIONS AND CAUTIONS

Managers can focus the team and show their support for the project by consideration of the following:

- Which functions are represented on the team and who is missing?

- The gap shown between where you are today and where you would like to be provides the emphasis needed on this QFD application.

- The project schedule can be used as a contract between team members.

- Remember, keep your brain in gear and do what is appropriate.

STOP AND REFLECT

This section sets the context for the project as a whole. The exercises identify critical tasks for the project team, assign responsibilities and completion dates, and determine which documents will serve as evidence of completion of critical steps. Like messenger RNA in the cell, the project flowchart and project schedule shape the overall design and set targets that call forth sequences of necessary actions to reach these targets. Without such a structure for the whole project, target dates slip, tasks are incomplete, old ways of doing things reassert themselves, and a new and self-organizing delivery system fails to emerge. In nature, design begins with the whole and the complexity of parts unfolds within the whole, thereby ensuring interconnectedness.

Chapter 6

Priority of Customer Segments

Upon completion of this chapter, you will be able to:

- Identify customer segments

- Prioritize customer segments

- Use the analytical hierarchy process (AHP)

In chapter 2, we presented a series of visual exercises and data that showed the world we routinely experience as a highly processed map. Presuppositions and embodied measures are incorporated into the map by the time the world appears to us (the disk with rectangle). The map is ordered to fit our expectations and embodied narratives (Ames's room and split-brain experiments), and we routinely fill in gaps in the map (blind spot). QFD includes tools that are designed to expand awareness beyond this habitual conditioning. We, like the cell, can expand our awareness by turning our attention to what is going on outside. The QFD process begins by identifying who the customers are and getting outside the organization to ask them what is important to them. What is uncovered is ranked and integrated into a new whole. This dance between divergent (expanding) and convergent (focusing) tools continues throughout the process. This chapter begins by expanding the team's awareness of customers and stakeholders.

WHO ARE THE CUSTOMERS?

Who should influence the design of your service? The QFD team begins by identifying customers and stakeholders. The goal is not only to identify who uses the service but also to identify who influences decisions as to whether or not to utilize the service. Cast a broad net to identify as many stakeholders and customers as possible. Identifying all stakeholders and their needs often identifies overlooked customer segments and the key needs for satisfying these customers. The process begins by identifying potential customers. Potential customers who are not identified will not have a voice in the design of the service. For this reason, the search for customer segments must be thorough. Steps 1 and 2 of QFD set a broad outline for goals of the service—the targets and values of the performance measures for these targets.

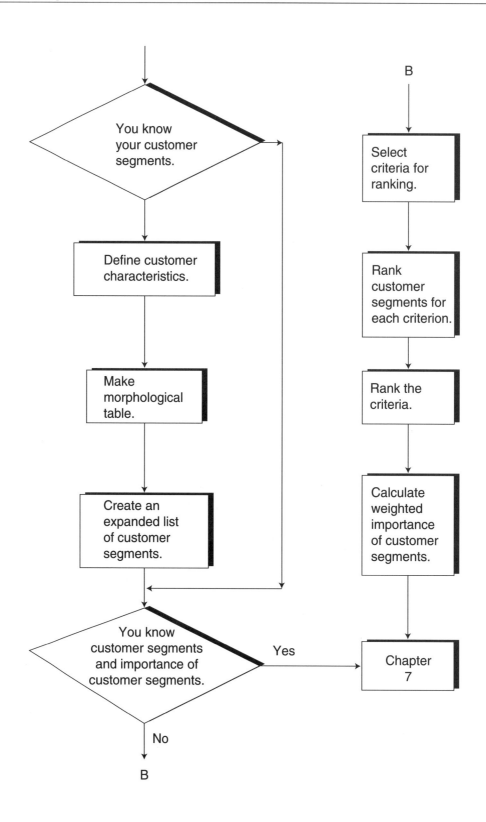

Capturing, ranking, and choosing which data to respond to is a function we all do more or less naturally and unconsciously every day. Sometimes our habits of doing so are effective and sometimes they are not. QFD attempts to make the semiautomatic actions implicit in our successful behaviors more explicit. In this section, we identify specific customers within the universe of potential customers, as well as different customer segments within the identified group. We also identify stakeholders, and we identify criteria for ranking customers/stakeholders in order of their importance to your organization.

The identity of the customer is not always readily apparent, nor is it agreed upon by all members of an organization. Like most healthcare providers in areas of the country where there has been high penetration of managed care, Rehab Concepts (a New England–based physical rehabilitation company providing services to injured workers) had come to see the customers as the insurer and the employer. These were the groups that paid the bills. Insurers and employers focus on getting injured employees back to work. After Rehab Concepts rediscovered the injured workers and their particular wants and needs, the organization became the preferred source for physical rehabilitation for industrial accidents in their market.

Many unintended consequences are the result of missing a customer segment or stakeholder in the initial product or service design. For example, hospitals typically do not focus on patient/customer needs during transport. Consequently, most hospitals provide less protection for the patient during the transit from the ambulance into the ER than trucking depots do for their cargo. Pharmaceutical organizations typically include patients, physicians, and pharmacists as their customers and stakeholders. Many of the pharmaceuticals that are ingested have a low rate of transfer from the gastrointestinal tract into the body. In communities where water comes from sources that include upstream sewage, commonly ingested pharmaceuticals such as estrogen and vitamin C are beginning to rise in the drinking water. In some cities in Germany, it may soon be possible for residents to get a daily minimum dose of vitamin C by drinking the city water. The community and the water utility were not considered as stakeholders in the pharmaceutical companies' processes.

Sometimes there are conflicts between purchaser and user. Some examples include:

- *Human/pet dog*—One dog-food manufacturer thought they considered everyone (veterinarians, nutritionists, trainers, breeders, and owners) in a new product. After a heavy introductory marketing campaign, the product sold out during the first month. The second month they sold nothing because the dogs would not eat the food.

- *Parent/child*—The same thing can happen when a parent buys the perfect food for their child who will not eat it.

- *Child/elderly parent*—The child buys medication or a device for the elderly parent (patient) who will not take or use it.

- *Employers/employees*—Employers and insurers want injured workers to return to work and stop expensive treatments as soon as they have overcome physical limitations from the injury that impede returning to work. As Rehab Concepts discovered, the employees are also concerned with regaining their functional capacities for recreational activities.

- *Purchaser/users*—The purchasing department gets a good buy on prepackaged procedure trays, such as those for lumbar punctures. However, physicians find some components difficult to use, so they do not use the trays.

The QFD team in our example did cast a broad net and identified a wide range of potential stakeholders (Figure 6.1).

EXERCISE 6.1

Use a brainstorming process to identify all individuals and organizations that can influence decisions to use or not use the service.

Morphological Table

Throughout the QFD process, there are tools and practices to *identify what may be missing*. A *morphological table* is one such tool. This table is used to expand awareness of customer segments and stakeholders. A morphological table creates a universe of all possible participants/customers and identifies the characteristics of each customer segment. Each particular customer segment may have different needs and demand different products and services. As an example of how a morphological table is constructed and used, consider an author of a murder mystery looking for a new story. Every mystery story has someone murdered, a means used, the killer, a motive, the location of the crime, the hero, and so on. These comprise the column headings, with specific possibilities for each listed in the columns. The morphological table in Figure 6.2 establishes the macro-model for a murder mystery story.

Out of this universe of possible combinations, the author chooses one characteristic from each column, shown as a shaded cell. The story characteristics shaded in the figure would have a homeless person electrocuted by a monk whose motive was revenge. The murder occurred at a dinner party, and the crime was solved by a teenager. These six characteristics define a story. A different set of characteristics would yield a different story.

Customers. Characteristics to identify customer segments for the customers in Figure 6.1 might include age, type of injury, time since injury, and whether the claim was in litigation or not. These become column headings for the morphological table (Figure 6.3).

Each of the details in the figure could become important characteristics for sorting individuals into customer segments. The 52-year-old manual laborer who sustained a head injury when he/she was crushed by a forklift (caused by a machine) one year earlier represents a different customer segment than the 60-year-old executive who strained his back (caused by the worker) while moving furniture yesterday. Each would have different needs and different demanded qualities to satisfy these needs.

The purpose of using the morphological table is to identify these different needs and thus the different services required to supply these needs. If a table does not demonstrate diversity, either the characteristics are wrong or there is only one customer group. One characteristic may be sufficient for sorting customers into segments, but as many as possible are needed to identify all possible customer segments. The best characteristics are mutually exclusive descriptors of the customer segments.

A point of caution: Do not confuse customer *characteristics* that are used to identify and *sort* customers into segments with *criteria* that will be used to *rank* the customer

CUSTOMERS	**Direct Consumers** Patients Over 65 Under 65 Family Members Over 65 Under 65
	Payers Medicare MediCal County Services % Charges Per Diem Capitated Workers' Compensation Insurers
	Referrals Agents Case Managers Physicians Families Skilled Nursing Facilities
	Physicians Treating Primary Others
	Employers Attorneys Plaintiff Defense

Figure 6.1. Customer segments. The team in the case example initially generated this list of possible customer segments and stakeholder segments.

	Murdered	Method	Killer	Motive	Location	Hero
1	Millionaire	Poison	Police	Passion	Yacht	Cat
2	Homeless	Gun	Lover	Hate	Camping	Butler
3	Child	Electrocution	Weight Lifter	Revenge	Dinner Party	Charlie Chan
4	Guru	Dart	Monk	Random	Hunting	Columbo
5	General	Arrow	Lawyer		Work	Teenager
6		Fear				

Figure 6.2. Morphological table for a mystery. Characteristics that describe a murder mystery are listed as column headings. Each combination of one element from each column creates a new story line.

	Age	Type of Workers	Type of Injury	Cause of Injury	Time since Injury	Level of Litigation
1	41–50	Executive	Hand	The Worker	0 year	None
2	51–60	Supervisor	Head	Machine	1 year	Just Started
3	61–70	Manual Laborer	Neck	Coworker	2 years	In Hearing
4	71–80		Back	Chemical	3 years	

Figure 6.3. Morphological table. The columns of the table identify characteristics that can be used to sort customers into segments. By selecting various combinations from the rows of the table, the team can expand its awareness of customer segments and potential customer segments.

segments in order of importance to your organization. This caution will become clear as we proceed.

Stakeholders. Developing a complete set of stakeholders requires a different process. For stakeholders, we look for different sources of influence, such as relationship, financial obligation, legal position, and so on. The morphological table shown in Figure 6.4 is from the case study. One possible segment is shown by the shaded cells. Since both customers and stakeholders have needs, both groups will be treated as and called customers in the QFD process from this point forward.

Identify Missing Segments. Using the same technique applied for the mystery novel, the QFD team can choose different combinations of characteristics from each column to identify unique customer segments. The goal is to identify any missing customer segments.

A worker's attorney has an ethical relationship to the worker, approaches the problems from the plaintiff's perspective, has a pro-worker bias, and relies on legal and regulatory language to understand and communicate. In the case example, the plaintiff attorneys were identified as a potential customer segment to focus on in the future.

EXERCISE 6.2

Identify three characteristics you can use to define the customer segments. Use these characteristics to build a morphological table and to expand the set of customers and potential customers. For an actual application, use whatever number of characteristics is relevant. Place these characteristics in a table and define them for two or three examples.

EXERCISE 6.3

Identify new customer segments. Which are important now, and which should be looked at in the future?

	Players	Financial Obligation	Legal Position	Preinjury Biases	Primary Language
1	None	None	None	None	Lay
2	Judges	Personal	Plaintiff	Pro-Worker	Medical
3	Employer	Regulatory	Defendant	Pro-Employer	Legal
4	Family	Ethical		Pro-Insurer	Political
5	Insurance Case Manager				
6	Representative				
7	Physician Treating				
8	Primary Care Physician				
9	Insurance Legal Clerk				
10	Worker's Attorneys				

Figure 6.4. Morphological table for stakeholders. The characteristics that can be used to identify stakeholders are listed as column headings, and examples are listed as entries.

STOP AND REFLECT

A beginning list of customer segments and stakeholders was generated. Characteristics of customers were identified. A morphological table was constructed to expand these lists and to identify segments within populations of customers and stakeholders.

Next a list of criteria will be generated to evaluate the importance of these segments to the project and the organization and will now explore tools to rank these segments and criteria.

DATA

The collected data are as key to any total quality management (TQM) project as data are for any study using the scientific method. Not all data contain the same amount of information. It is important to understand the quality of information embedded in any set of data. Not all numbers contain the same depth of information. We will review four types of measures that capture and organize signals from the environment into meaningful data. These are nominal, ordinal, interval, and ratio data.

Nominal Data
Nominal data is categorical data. For example, ICD-9 codes are used to classify diagnoses. A hip fracture is 820, a fractured neck of the humerus is 812, and a stroke is 436.

There is no meaning in the result of taking these categorical numbers and averaging them. The result is nonsense. Nominal data is mathematically sound for counting and calculating the mode. The mode is the number (diagnostic group) that occurs most frequently.

Ordinal Data

Ordinal data denotes a position in a hierarchy. The order of the numbers has a significant meaning. The interval between the numbers does not. For example many hospitals use a five-point satisfaction scale, where 5 is "excellent" and 1 is "poor". A survey rating of 4 is higher than a survey rating of 2, but the rating of 4 is not twice the rating of 2. The median is the middle number for a data set and has meaning. Calculating means (averages) is not appropriate.

Interval Data

Interval data denotes a position in a hierarchy, and the distance between positions also has meaning. With this measure, the interval between 3 and 6 is the same as the interval between 6 and 9. All three of the measures of central tendency (mean, median, and mode) can be used.

Any measurement system with an artificial zero point provides interval data. Body temperature using the Fahrenheit or Celsius scales provides interval data. The average, median, and mode all have mathematical meaning and practical use. Calculating the standard deviation to understand the variation in body temperature is also mathematically correct and medically useful. Calculating ratios, however, is not mathematically sound. A patient with a 102-degree temperature is not 2 percent hotter than when they had a 100-degree temperature. The number 102 is 2 percent higher but not 2 percent hotter. Neither ratios nor multiplication and division between data points are meaningful with the interval scale data.

Ratio Data

Ratio data scales include absolute zero. We tend to treat all numbers as ratio data because so many numbers in our life are. Some examples are length, area, volume, time, counting, and pressure. With ratio data, calculating the mode, median, and mean (average) are all meaningful, as are multiplication and division between data.

Pulse and blood pressure are examples of ratio data. You may remember in college chemistry or physics that the Fahrenheit and Celsius temperature readings were changed to Rankin or Kelvin, respectively, to make ratio comparisons. Ratio data contains more information than interval data; interval data contains more information than ordinal data; and ordinal data contains more information than nominal data.

SCALES

Most human assessments about needs and satisfaction are captured by having people rank preferences. Most of the data is ordinal data. The category and order within the category are meaningful. The "distance" between categories is not measured. For our work in QFD, we will be using four types of ranking scales to capture and interpret data from the customer: five-point scales, an asymmetrical three-point scale, distribution of 100 points, and nine-point scales for pairwise comparisons.

Five-Point Scales

The 1–5 Likert scale is very commonly used in surveys, as reflected in the case study (Figure 4.3). These scales provide ordinal data. Two five-point scales used in Figure 4.3 follow:

5	Very strongly matters	5	Excellent
6	Strongly matters	4	Above average
7	Matters	3	Average
2	Somewhat matters	2	Below average
1	Does not matter	1	Poor

Research by Thomas Saaty (1993) indicates that a nine-point scale is more repeatable than a five-, seven-, eight-, or ten-point scale. However, a nine-point scale is more of a challenge for the customer than the five-point, and five-point scales are still the most commonly used.

Asymmetrical Three-Point Scales

This scale is used to correlate rows and columns in the matrix tools:

● Strong

◐ Medium

○ Weak

Distribution of 100 Points

Customers are asked to weight different characteristics by distributing 100 points between the characteristics. The distribution of 100 points is used in some marketing studies. Prior to designing a new clinic, a company might ask members of a customer segment to rank selected aspects of the services of a clinic. For example, a questionnaire might ask the future customers to distribute 100 points between location, hours of operation, and services offered to determine their relative importance. A sample response might be

Location	50
Hours open	30
Services	20

Nine-Point Scales and Pairwise Comparisons

Nine-Point Scale
9. Extreme importance
8. Between 9 and 7
7. Very strong importance
6. Between 7 and 5
5. Strong importance
4. Between 5 and 3
3. Moderate importance
2. Between 3 and 1
1. Equal importance

The pairwise comparison approach used in this text is called the analytical hierarchy process (AHP) (Saaty 1993). Psychological studies have shown that humans have difficulty comparing more than seven items and perform best when comparing two items in direct pairwise comparisons. We have no difficulty judging the relative weights between two stones, but we are not very good at ranking the 61 demanded qualities identified in the case study. However, by grouping data and using Saaty's method of a nine-point scale and full pairwise comparisons, we can create ratio rankings for all of our demanded qualities.

RANKING CUSTOMER SEGMENTS

Not all customer segments and stakeholders are equally important. If the relative importance of one customer segment to another is not obvious, then a formal ranking process with criteria for ranking must be used. To do so effectively, the criteria for ranking must also be ranked.

In the case study, the customer segments were not formally ranked. It is common when beginning to use the QFD process that the most important customer segments are obvious. However, a formal process of ranking criteria used to rank customer segments is the central building block to the QFD process. Often, organizations assume they know which customers are the most important without having explicitly stated criteria supporting their belief. When criteria are stated, the relative importance of the criteria is often missing.

Sometimes customer segments are clear as in the case example. When they are not, it is easy to see how unsupported assumptions lead to self-fulfilling prophecies. These assumptions continue to create a future that is based on and looks like the past. If customer segments or ways of accomplishing a particular task are selected without first making the criteria for selection explicit, you produce choices that are not supported. Consider the following case.

Prior to May 1999, in the state of New Hampshire, each town and city was responsible for funding the education of its students. A small amount of supplemental funding came from the state lottery. In 1997, the New Hampshire State Supreme Court declared that the existing system for funding public education was unconstitutional because the state was not funding education equitably for all students. The state had until April 1, 1999, to institute a new method to fund public education. Initial discussions were to amend the state constitution, but this did not occur.

During the first quarter of 1999, the public began to hear of a number of alternative plans for funding education. At first, weekly, and then daily, news broadcasts and newspaper stories discussed the various options. There was no discussion about how the legislature would rank the options, only discussions of how many votes each option appeared to have.

When there is only one clear criterion, it is easy to decide which option is better. Would you prefer winning $1000 or $5000? That is not a difficult choice. Deciding whether to fund education via income tax or property tax is not so clear. This is the problem of deciding what is important. QFD uses the strategy of trying to make explicit the unspoken criteria that underlie such decisions.

Once the criteria are explicit, it becomes obvious that the criteria are not all equally important. When criteria are agreed upon, the relative importance of each criterion needs to be ranked. Once the definition of the criteria and their relative relationships are agreed upon, the performance of each option for each criterion can be determined and composite scores for each of the options can be calculated based on how well they satisfy the agreed-upon criteria. Usually this process expands the awareness of the participants, and the results are more easily accepted than the results of traditional meetings and discussions.

If the decision makers do not like the option with the highest score, there are several possible explanations. Either the agreed-upon criteria are incorrectly ranked, or the performance of the options for each agreed-upon criterion are incorrect. When decision makers do not like the option with the highest score, it is often psychological inertia that is trapping people in their old paradigm. For example, a long-standing mantra opposing broad-based taxes is a root cause for the argument against options that distribute the funding burden for education over the whole state.

In New Hampshire, the default method for the community was the casting of ballots by the legislature, where each legislator used his or her own personal criteria when voting. In mid-May, the legislature somehow decided to have a broad-based property tax to help fund education in poorer towns. There was little community understanding about how, why, and what criteria were used to choose this method. Within one week, a lawsuit challenging the decision was filed.

Returning to the case example, Figure 6.1 shows that the team did cast a broad net for potential stakeholders/customers. The challenge to the team by the organization was to institute changes that would improve their service such that the volume of referrals would increase. Early in the project, the team generated a list of potential criteria that could be used to rank customer segments by order of importance. The criteria include possibilities and barriers to increasing referrals to the service. Four of these criteria included:

- Potential for repeat referrals

- Difficulty to contact

- Ease to satisfy

- Word-of-mouth referrals (i.e., customer-to-customer marketing)

EXERCISE 6.4

Generate several criteria appropriate for ranking your customer segments.

The criteria for identifying important customer segments must be clearly defined and understood by the team. Make notes of the discussion supporting team decisions. This may seem inordinately detailed and laborious, but keep in mind that this part of our process is equal to 95 percent of a cell's *stimulus-response time*—the time the cell invests in processing the implications of stimuli before it selects targets and moves into action. Defining customer segments requires defining and determining customer characteristics for sorting. Understanding the relative importance between customer segments requires criteria to rank these customer segments.

For some new initiates to QFD, the ranking tools in this chapter may seem to be the most difficult in the text to grasp. This material does, however, represent the direction in which the competition is going (Palmer 1999). These concepts and tools are key to identifying what is important.

The following is an example of the steps used to rank customer segments. In these examples, customer segments will be ranked for the first criterion the team listed in the case example *potential for repeat referrals.* There are three types of criteria used for ranking data:

- Larger-is-better ratio data

- Smaller-is-better ratio data

- Target is best; no ratio data is available (When ratio data is not available, the AHP is used.)

Because the case study involved redesigning an existing service, these steps were not carried out. The following illustrates sample rankings for these three data types, using development of new services for acutely injured workers as a hypothetical example. To build a network providing services to injured workers, an early step is to search for workers who have been recently injured. Each of the three types of data is presented separately. In an actual problem, some combination of data types usually exists.

Normalizing Larger-Is-Better Data

Data for ranking options or customer segments for a particular criteria may be available from trade journals, industry associations, or local business organizations. Data on injuries in a community, region, or state are often available. In one metropolitan area of two million residents, there are approximately 1,100,000 workers and 96,000 employers. Only 81 are publicly traded companies. The largest employers in the community are hospital systems. Most people work in small businesses. Assume that there are 80,000 new work-related injuries requiring medical evaluation per year. Assume also that, of these, 12,000 are referred by the injured workers themselves; 60,000 are referred by employers; and 8,000 are referred by insurance case managers. This is ratio data and can be used to rank the relative importance of each of these segments in referring repeat business for services. The data is a count, and the counts must be normalized (Figure 6.5). For a service being directed toward newly injured workers and using the criteria *repeat referrals,* employers would be 7.5 times more important than insurance case managers ($75 \div 10 = 7.5$).

EXERCISE 6.5

If this is a practice or learning exercise, select three criteria to be used for practice. If one of the criteria is *larger-is-better,* imagine that ratio data is available to you. Build a table as in Figure 6.5. If this is an actual project, use collected data.

Normalizing Smaller-Is-Better Data

A trade magazine with an article about the number of sales calls necessary to actually generate a referral for each particular customer segment exemplifies another type of ratio data, *smaller-is-better.* This data must be normalized to determine relative importance. The table in Figure 6.6 shows the number of calls to each segment to generate referrals. Assume the number of calls is 100 for workers, 10 for employers and 6 for individual case managers. The fewer the calls, the more desirable the customer. The reciprocal of each datum must be calculated before finding the normalized percent (the reciprocal is 1/datum). Therefore, the reciprocal of 100 for the *worker* is 0.01. The total of all the reciprocals is 0.277. This total is used to calculate the percent importance for each customer.

Normalizing Larger-Is-Better Patio Data (For newly injured)				
Repeat Referrals	**Injured Workers**	**Employers**	**Insurance Case Managers**	**Total**
Raw Data	12,000	60,000	8,000	80,000
% of Total	15	75	10	100

Figure 6.5. Normalizing larger-is-better ratio data. Raw data is obtained as counts, which are translated into ratio data.

Normalizing Smaller-Is-Better Ratio Data (For newly Injured)				
Ease to Contact	**Workers**	**Employers**	**Insurance Case Managers**	**Total**
Raw Data	100	10	6	—
Inverted Data	0.01	0.1	0.167	0.277
%	3.61	36.10	60.29	100.00

Figure 6.6. Normalizing smaller-is-better ratio data. Here, the fewer the better, so before normalizing the data, 1/datum is calculated and then expressed as a percent of total.

The value of the inverted data for each segment (e.g., 0.01 for workers) is divided by this total (0.277) and multiplied by 100 to yield a relative percent importance.

$$(0.01/0.277) \times 100 = 3.61\%$$

For the criteria *ease to contact,* the insurance case managers are almost twice as important as the employers.

EXERCISE 6.6

Reword one of your criteria to make it a *smaller-is-better* type. Create some ratio data to suit this criterion. Replicate the calculation in Figure 6.6. If this is an actual project, use the collected data.

Analytical Hierarchy Process

When ratio data is not available, the team uses pairwise comparisons and the AHP process. The AHP process works with ratio data. If the data are not ratios, they are converted to ratio data by using paired comparisons. Supported by 30 years of research, AHP uses pairwise comparisons to enable decision making by considering many factors in seemingly complex, nonstructured situations (Saaty 1993). Consider the AHP process to be like trying to find the relative weight among pebbles in a group of pebbles

Ease to Satisfy	Injured Workers	Employers	Insurance Case Managers
Injured Workers			
Employers			
Insurance Case Managers			
Total			

Figure 6.7. Matrix table for pairwise comparisons. Set up a matrix table for *ease to satisfy* by entering customer segments in both columns and rows to yield a customer segment versus customer segment matrix table.

from heaviest to lightest without having access to a scale for ounces or grams. The process begins by comparing the weight of one pebble to another pebble to determine which is heavier (ordinal) and by how much (interval). This process is carried out for all the pebbles, yielding a relative ranking of all the pebbles to each other. Then the "scaler weight" of individual pebbles can be divided by the "total scaler weights" for all the pebbles giving a ratio or relative weight of each part to the whole.

Pairwise Comparisons

Set Up Matrix Table: First set up a customer segment versus customer segment matrix table for the criterion Ease to Satisfy (Figure 6.7).

Start Pairwise Comparisons: Comparisons are made between each of the rows and columns. Each row of the table is compared to the column by asking the question, "Is the row more important than the column?" If the answer is yes, how much more important is the row compared to the column? Use a nine-point comparison scale as defined in the following box.

Nine-Point Scale

9. Extreme importance: the evidence favoring the row is of the highest possible order or affirmation.
8. Between 7 and 9.
7. Very strong importance: the row is strongly favored, and its dominance is demonstrated in practice.
6. Between 5 and 7.
5. Strong importance: experience and judgment strongly favor the row over the column.
4. Between 3 and 5.
3. Moderate importance: experience and judgment slightly favor the row over the column.
2. Between 1 and 3.
1. Equal importance: the row and column have the same impact upon the higher order need.

Ease to Satisfy	Injured Workers	Employers	Insurance Case Managers
Injured Workers	1	/	
Employers			
Insurance Case Managers			
Total			

Figure 6.8. Comparison matrix continued. Comparisons are made between the rows and columns. Each row of the table is compared to the column by asking the question, "Is the row more important than the column?" using the nine-point scale. If the answer is *Yes*, the value from the nine-point scale is entered; if *No*, a forward slash for the divide operation is entered.

Pairwise comparisons can be made on the basis of importance, preference, or likelihood:

- *Importance* is used for comparing one criterion with another.

- *Preference* is used for comparing alternatives.

- *Likelihood* is used for comparing the probability of outcomes and is appropriate for criteria of alternatives.

The weights can be either verbal or numerical. When working with customers, however, the verbal form of the nine-point scale should be used rather than numbers.

The value from the scale is placed in that cell of the matrix. If the answer to the question "Is the row more important then the column?" is no, a forward slash (/), for the divide operation, is placed in the cell (Figure 6.8). In the matrix, the row *Injured workers* is equal to the column *Injured workers* and therefore is given a rating of *1*.

Moving left to right in the same row, the team assesses *Employers* as more likely to be *easy to satisfy* than *Injured workers,* so a forward slash is placed in the cell. The same is the case for the rest of the cells in the row.

Next, *Employers* were assessed as strongly more likely to be *easy to satisfy* than *Injured workers,* and a *5* was placed in the cell. This process continues until all rows are compared to columns (Figure 6.9).

Activities for the "Less Than" Cells in the Rows: Now the cells with the forward slash (division symbol) must be evaluated. The cell representing the team's assessment for the *Employers* versus *Injured workers* indicated that *Employers* are strongly more likely to be *easy to satisfy,* 5. The highlighted cell for *Injured workers* versus *Employers* must be 1/5 to be consistent (Figure 6.10). That is, *Injured workers* are 1/5 as likely as *Employers* to be *easy to satisfy.* The rest of the matrix is completed in a similar manner. When the matrix is completed, a diagonal of 1 to 1 relationships is present where identical rows and columns intersect. The cells below and to the left of the diagonal are the reciprocal of the cells above and to the right.

Ease to Satisfy	Injured Workers	Employers	Insurance Case Managers
Injured Workers	1	/	/
Employers	5	1	/
Insurance Case Managers	9	5	1
Total			

Figure 6.9. Comparison matrix continued. The comparisons started in Figure 6.8 are continued until all the *Yes* responses have values.

Ease to Satisfy	Injured Workers	Employers	Insurance Case Managers
Injured Workers	1	1/5	1/9
Employers	5	1	1/5
Insurance Case Managers	9	5	1
Total			

Figure 6.10. Comparison matrix continued. Here, values for the "less than" cells in the rows are entered as reciprocals.

Consistency Checks: Consistency checks are made to ensure the reliability of the ratios. For example, if *Employers* are 5 times more likely to be *easy to satisfy* than *Injured workers* and *Insurance case managers* are 5 times more likely to be *easy to satisfy* than *Employers,* then for the table to be consistent *Insurance case managers* must be 10 times more likely to be *easy to satisfy* than *Injured workers.* The team had entered a 9 in this cell indicating the ranking was internally consistent. [At the time this book was written, there was software available for doing the mathematical calculations and checking for consistency. A demo version is available on the webpage: www.expertchoice.com (We have no financial relation to expert choice.)]

EXERCISE 6.7

Select one of the customer criterion for which the team must use AHP to rank importance, performance, or likelihood. Build a comparison matrix for the criterion. Assign ratings using the nine-point scale as described in the preceding paragraphs.

	Reciprocol	
9	Extremely	0.111
8		0.125
7	Very Strongly	0.143
6		0.167
5	Strongly	0.200
4		0.250
3	Moderately	0.333
2		0.500
1	Equally	1.000

Ease to Satisfy	Injured Workers	Employers	Insurance Case Managers
Injured Workers	1.00	0.20	0.11
Employers	5.00	1.00	0.20
Insurance Case Managers	9.00	5.00	1.00
Total	15.00	6.20	1.31

Figure 6.11. Comparison matrix converting to decimal data. Here, the values initially entered in the comparison matrix are converted to decimal form. The columns are then summed.

Converting to Decimal Data

Convert Data to Decimals: The decimal equivalent is found for all the fractions calculated (Figure 6.11). The reciprocals of the weights are given in the box at the top of this page.

Total Columns: The columns are then added for the total weight of each column (see Figure 6.11)

Normalizing Data

Normalize Cells: Normalizing data is accomplished by dividing the value in each cell in Figure 6.11 by the total value of the column within which the cell lies (Figure 6.12). For example, the first cell in Figure 6.11 is *Injured workers* versus *Injured Workers* with a value of 1. The total for the column is 15.

$$1/15 = 0.067$$

This value is placed in the corresponding cells in Figure 6.12.

Sum the Rows: Each row is summed. If the calculations are correct and consistent, the figure for the sum of the rows in each column equals the number of segments (Figure 6.13).

Ease to Satisfy	Injured Workers	Employers	Insurance Case Managers	Total	%
Injured Workers	0.067	0.032	0.084		
Employers	0.333	0.161	0.153		
Insurance Case Managers	0.600	0.806	0.763		
Total	1.000	1.000	1.000		

Figure 6.12. Comparison matrix continued: normalizing data and calculating weights. The value entered into each cell of the column in Figure 6.1 is converted to a fraction of the total weight for the column by dividing the value of the cell by the total of the column.

Ease to Satisfy	Injured Workers	Employers	Insurance Case Managers	Total	Averaged Expressed as %
Injured Workers	0.067	0.032	0.084	0.183	6.1
Employers	0.333	0.161	0.153	0.647	21.6
Insurance Case Managers	0.600	0.806	0.763	2.170	72.3
Total	1.000	1.000	1.000	3.000	100

Figure 6.13. Comparison matrix continued: normalizing data and calculating weights. The average for each row is calculated by summing the row and dividing by the number of columns in the row, in this case three. The data can be expressed as a percentage for ease of comparison and visibility.

Compute the Average for Each Category in the Row: Finally, the average for each row is calculated (Figure 6.13). This is the total for the row divided by the number of data, in this case three.[1] Since this average also describes the relative weights of the respective rows to the whole, it can be expressed as a percentage for visibility and ease of communication.

The criteria *Ease to satisfy* was approximately 3.3 times more important for the *Insurance case managers* than for *Employers:*

$$72.1/21.6 = 3.3$$

---

[1]Without going into the details as to why this value approximates the Eigen vector of the matrix table.

Criteria	PRR	EC	ES	Total	%
PRR	1	7	3		
EC	1/7	1	1		
ES	1/3	1	1		
Total					

Figure 6.14. Pairwise comparison matrix for criteria. Each row of the table is compared to the column by asking the question, "Is the row more important than the column?" If the answer is *Yes,* by how much on the nine-point scale is entered. The matrix is then completed by entering reciprocals in the appropriate columns.

EXERCISE 6.8

Complete all the calculations, as shown in Figure 6.13, to determine which segments are preferred for the selected criterion.

STOP AND REFLECT

Four types of data were discussed: normal, ordinal, interval, and ratio. The four primary scales used in QFD to capture and organize data were presented: five-point scales, asymmetrical three-point scales, distribution of 100 points, and nine-point scales for pairwise comparisons.

The customer segments were ranked for each criteria. When ratio data are available, they are normalized and the results are used in ranking. When ratio data are not available, AHP is used to generate ratio data. Next, the relative importance of each criteria is determined using AHP.

RANKING CRITERIA

AHP is used to rank the importance of the criteria: *potential for repeat referrals (PRR), ease of contact (EC),* and *ease to satisfy (ES).* Pairwise comparisons are done to complete the matrix (Figure 6.14).
Data are converted to decimal form (Figure 6.15).
Data are normalized, rows are summed, and averages are computed (Figure 6.16).
Potential for repeat referrals (68.6 percent) was weighted as the most important criteria.

RANKING CUSTOMER SEGMENTS
WITH RANKED CRITERIA

Finally, the customer segments previously ranked for each criterion need to be weighted by the importance of the criteria used to rank them. The data generated for customer importance and for the criteria are entered into a weighted importance table of customer segments (Figure 6.17). The first two columns contain *criteria* and *importance of criteria,* respectively. These two columns are the criteria and the relative

Criteria	PRR	EC	ES	Total	%
PRR	1.00	7.00	3.00		
EC	0.14	1.00	1.00		
ES	0.33	1.00	1.00		
Total	1.47	9.00	5.00		

Figure 6.15. Comparison matrix: decimal form. The values for the cells in Figure 6.14 are converted to decimal form.

Criteria	PRR	EC	ES	Total	%
PRR	0.680	0.777	0.600	2.057	68.6
EC	0.095	0.111	0.200	0.406	13.6
ES	0.224	0.111	0.200	0.535	17.8
Total	1.000	1.000	1.000	2.998	100.0

Figure 6.16. Comparison matrix: normalization of data. Each of the values in the cells is then expressed as a fraction of the total value of the column, the rows added, and the average calculated and expressed as a percent.

weights of importance of the criteria from Figure 6.16 (see Figure 6.18, a summary figure). The next three columns in Figure 6.17 are the "raw" importance of each customer segment for each criterion. These entries come from the *normalizing larger-is-better ratio data for repeat referrals* (Figure 6.5), *normalizing smaller-is-better ratio data for Ease to contact* (Figure 6.6), and the *pairwise AHP comparison for Ease to satisfy* (Figure 6.13).

These raw data have not yet taken into account differences in importance of the criteria themselves. The importance of each customer segment is adjusted by the weight of the selected criterion. This is explained using the shaded cell in Figure 6.17.

The weight of the criterion *Potential for repeat referrals (PRR)* as calculated using AHP is 0.680 (Figure 6.16). The importance weight for *Injured workers* for this criterion was calculated as 0.150. The weighted importance for *Injured workers* is the product of the two, 0.102.

Customer segment importance weight × Criteria weight
= Weighted preference (0.150 × 0.680 = 0.102)

The remaining weighted preferences are calculated in the same manner. Columns under weighted preferences are summed. The sum of all the weighted preferences for each customer segment gives the composite preference for that segment relative to the group of

		Unweighted			Weighted		
Criteria	**Import.**	**Injured Workers**	**Employers**	**Ins. Case Managers**	**Injured Workers**	**Employers**	**Ins. Case Managers**
PRR	0.680	0.150	0.750	0.100	0.102	0.51	0.068
EC	0.095	0.036	0.361	0.603	0.0034	0.0343	0.0573
ES	0.224	0.061	0.216	0.723	0.0137	0.0484	0.1620
Total	1.000				0.1191	0.5927	0.2872

Figure 6.17. Weighted importance of customer segments. This matrix is a criteria versus customer segment matrix. The importance ratings of criteria are entered into the first column, and the importance of those criteria to each customer segment (raw preference) is entered into the next three columns. The raw preferences are then weighted by multiplying the raw weight for the customer importance by the criteria weight. The columns, customer segments, are then added such that the relative weights for the customer segments are obtained.

criteria. When the table is complete, the total weighted importance for the three customer segments should equal 1, and the data can be displayed as a percentage (for example 59.27) or as decimal data. When the customer segments are ranked using criteria that are also used for newly injured workers, the *Employers* are the preferred customer segment.

STOP AND REFLECT

Not all customer segments are equally important in developing a new business. A morphological table was developed to expand organizational awareness and to identify various customer segments. Criteria for ranking the different customer segments were identified and clarified. The importance of each customer segment relative to the criteria was then determined. The criteria themselves were ranked. The ranked criteria were then used to weight the importance of customer segments relative to the criteria.

In this example, ratio data was available for the criteria *Potential for repeat referrals* and *Ease of contact*. This ratio data was used to weight these criteria and rank the customer segments relative to that criteria (Figure 6.5 and Figure 6.6, respectively). No ratio data was available for *Ease to satisfy*. For this criterion, the AHP with pairwise comparisons using a nine-point scale was used by the team to generate ratio data for ranking the customer segments (Figure 6.13).

Ratio data available from the environment is preferable for ranking criteria. When this information is not available, AHP is used to capture the collective experience and wisdom of the team for ranking both customer segments and criteria.

Figure 6.17 gives a ranking of customer importance for criteria and the weights of the criteria. How this all flows together is shown in Figure 6.18. Results of the activities to rank criteria were entered into a composite weighted importance of customer segments table as ratio data that is decimal data (Figure 6.16 in Figure 6.18). The "raw" (non-weighted) preferences for customer segments relative to each criteria were also entered

Figure 6.5. Normalizing larger-is-better ratio data.

Repeat Referrals	Injured Workers	Employers	Insurance Case Managers	Total
Raw Data	12,000	60,000	8,000	80,000
%	15	75	10	100

Figure 6.6. Normalizing smaller-is-better ratio data.

Ease to Contact	Workers	Employers	Insurance Case Managers	Total
Raw Data	100	10	6	—
Inverted Data	0.01	0.1	0.167	0.277
%	3.61	36.10	60.29	100.00

Figure 6.16. Comparison matrix: normalization of data.

Criteria	PRR	EC	ES	Total	%
PRR	0.680	0.777	0.600	2.057	68.6
EC	0.095	0.111	0.200	0.406	13.6
ES	0.224	0.111	0.200	0.535	17.8
Total	1.000	1.000	1.000	2.998	100.0

Figure 6.13. Comparison matrix continued.

Ease to Satisfy	Injured Workers	Employers	Insurance Case Managers	Total	Averaged Expressed as %
Injured Workers	0.067	0.032	0.084	0.183	6.1
Employers	0.333	0.161	0.153	0.647	21.6
Insurance Case Managers	0.600	0.806	0.763	2.170	72.3
Total	1.000	1.000	1.000	3.000	100

Figure 6.17. Weighted importance of customer segments.

Criteria	Import.	Injured Workers	Employ-ers	Ins. Case Managers	Injured Workers	Employ-ers	Ins. Case Managers
PRR	0.680	0.150	0.750	0.100	0.102	0.51	0.068
EC	0.095	0.036	0.361	0.603	0.0034	0.0343	0.0573
ES	0.224	0.061	0.216	0.723	0.0137	0.0484	0.1620
Total	1.000				0.1191	0.5927	0.2872

Figure 6.18. Putting it all together. This figure shows how the parts calculated throughout this section come together and are used to generate a clear picture of cutstomers and the importance of different customer segments.

as ratio data (Figures 6.5, 6.6, and 6.13 in Figure 6.18). A composite weighted preference for each customer segment, which includes the criteria importance, was then calculated by summing the columns (Figure 6.17 in Figure 6.18). For the new service for injured workers, *Employers* were identified as the most important customer segment.

In the case example presented in chapter 4, AHP was used for the customer segments for each criteria. The ranking for *Potential for repeat referrals (PRR)* is shown in Figure 6.16. Figure 6.19 shows the process in a spreadsheet format rather than as a series of tables. The first four columns contain the pairwise comparisons using the nine-point scale. The next four columns are decimal data, and the third set of four columns shows the normalized data. The rows are summed and then averaged to show the percentage importance.

In the case example, the goal was to increase referrals. The important customer segment was identified at this point in the process, and the team stopped here. If the process was continued, the customers would be ranked for each criteria and the criteria would be ranked, as shown in Figures 6.14 to 6.16. The resulting data would be placed in a Weighted Importance of Customer Segments Table (Figure 6.19). Having now identified which customer segments are most important to the organization, in Chapter 7 we will look at tools to identify what is important to these customer segments. Most acute injuries are referred directly from an employer to a healthcare provider. Most chronic problems, such as in the case example, are referred by insurance case managers to providers.

Discussion of Outcome

To anyone who is familiar with work injuries, the results produced by this example should be no surprise. Most acute injuries are referred directly from an employer to a healthcare provider. Most chronic and complex problems are referred by an insurance case manager to providers. However, the point of the example was to see how AHP works. If your organizational team is unfamiliar with what criteria you use to select and compare customer segments, this process will help generate consensus and consistency in interpreting your data. You can use AHP to prioritize customers, identify which of the many challenges facing the organization you will choose as the more important to work on, or purchase your next computer system. The power and value of AHP in ranking alternatives for complex situations (for example, which of 61 qualities demanded by customers are the most important) are addressed in a subsequent chapter.

SUGGESTIONS AND CAUTIONS

When in the Process Is It Best to Rank the Criteria?

The example in this chapter compared the customer segments for each of the criteria and then ranked the criteria (Figure 6.20). The advantage of this sequence is that the criteria become clarified during the discussions for ranking the customer segments. The ranking of the criteria is then based on a sound understanding of the criteria. The advantage of ranking the criteria first occurs when one of the criteria is so much more critical than the others for ranking the customer segments that the others are of no consequence. This happened for the project team potential for *repeat referrals* represented 68.6 percent of the value for customer segments (Figure 6.15). Since this was so significant and addressing this issue would be a breakthrough in thinking, only this criterion was used.

If you rank the criteria first, the team not uncommonly realizes during the subsequent ranking of the customer segments for each criterion that the definition of criteria

PRR	Insurers	Physicians	Injured Workers	Attorneys	Insurers	Physicians	Injured Workers	Attorneys	Insurers	Physicians	Injured Workers	Attorneys	Row Sums	%
Insurers	1	5	9	3	1	5	9	3	0.610	0.694	0.450	0.577	2.331	58.28
Physicians	1/5	1	5	1	0.2	1	5	1	0.122	0.139	0.250	0.192	0.703	17.58
Injured Workers	1/9	1/5	1	1/5	0.11	0.2	1	0.2	0.067	0.028	0.050	0.038	0.183	4.58
Plaintiff Attorneys	1/3	1	5	1	0.33	1	5	1	0.201	0.139	0.250	0.192	0.782	19.56
					1.64	7.2	20	5.2	1	1	1	1	4.000	100.00

Figure 6.19. AHP rankings from the case example. Here, the data is shown in one table using a spreadsheet instead of a series of matrix tables.

106

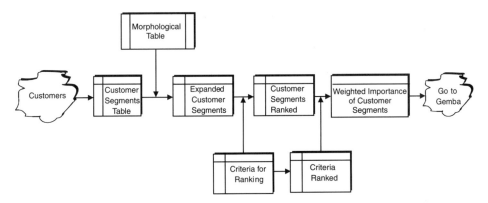

Figure 6.20. Summary flowchart. This flowchart shows how the sections and tools used in AHP are interconnected.

was not clear and new formulations of the criteria are made. It is now necessary to rerank the criteria.

In the case example in chapter 4, none of the criteria had ratio data for the case. The AHP process would have to be used for ranking the customer segments for each criterion. The final integration of the ranking of the criteria and customer segments for each criterion would be completed as in the example in this chapter.

AHP

AHP, like any ranking system, works if the items being compared are of the same order of magnitude. Comparing the brightness of the sun to a candle is not an appropriate comparison, nor is it necessary since the answer is obviously the sun.

The customer may tire of comparing all pairs of combinations for the list of items to be ranked. Nevertheless, the precision of the AHP process is well worth the effort. Practitioners and competitors evolve toward full pairwise comparisons as they become more experienced in capturing and assessing data. AHP has been used in a variety of applications, from selecting the location of an airport in Saudi Arabia, to selecting organizational development projects for the coming year (Palmer 1999).

You may have noticed in Figure 6.19 that only the odd numbers appear for the nine-point scale. Using the full nine points is recommended. This was the team's first QFD project; and, because of the process and the amount of debate over some items, the facilitator preferentially used 1, 3, 5, and 9 for weighting importance, likelihood, or preference. This strategy was chosen to reduce the time and debate around using the full nine-point scale.

When working with customers or teams and AHP, consensus is used to settle rankings. If consensus cannot be reached, a geometric mean is calculated for all answers and that value is used. A geometric mean is calculated by taking the nth (in this case, 4th) root of the product of all responses for the example:

$$\sqrt[4]{4 \times 2 \times 5 \times 2} = 3$$

The geometric mean is more appropriate than an arithmetic average. For example, if one customer feels that item X is twice as important as Y, but the second believes that item

X is half as important as *Y*, the arithmetic average would give *X* as 1.25 as much importance as *Y*. On the other hand, the geometric mean would give 1, showing that *X* and *Y* are equally important.

STOP AND REFLECT

Recall that 95 percent of the work the cell spends responding to perturbations from the environment involves processing the perturbations and transcribing (projecting) targets for the future (Figure 3.4). This section describes the preliminary work of QFD. It prepares the team to capture information about the customer's demands from the customer's environment. When done well, the tools in this section have already enhanced the team's awareness of its customers and have likely uncovered and either confirmed or rejected some preexisting assumption.

Some organizations find that prioritization of their customers provides enough new insights upon which to act. They do not continue with the QFD process. Instead, they return to the traditional design process without additional input from QFD. For the purpose of learning and for those continuing on the journey of change, the next chapter takes a detailed look at customer needs and desires.

Chapter 7

Understanding Your Customer

Upon completing this chapter, you will be able to:

- Map the environment where your service is used

- Build a high-level flowchart of how your service fits into your customer's environment

- Expand the list of customer-stated needs

- Sort the customer-stated needs into demanded qualities, performance measures, functions, and tasks

- Determine natural clusters of demanded qualities

- Determine the hierarchical importance of demanded qualities

CUSTOMER ENVIRONMENTS

The goal of the QFD tools described in this chapter is to enhance the organization and the team's understanding of customer needs, wants, and expectations. In many manufacturing sectors as well as in some service industries, organizations actually do go out into the customer's environments. People from a design team may actually work in the customer's organization for a period of months. Understanding the context in which the customer uses your service requires the expenditure of resources very early in the design process.

In the case study presented in chapter 4, the QFD team developed a high-level process map of the customer's interface with organizational services as the team interviewed customers in the field. Figure 7.1 is an overview of their customer's process. It is presented to show how the team's particular services fit into the customer's overall process. The first row of functions centers around treating injuries; the second row shows constraining unnecessary care; and the third row shows dispute resolution. The QFD team in chapter 4 was charged with improving the process for multidisciplinary evaluations, shown by the darker shaded functions (B in Figure 7.1). These shaded blocks are the services the QFD organization provides. Details of the process outlined in Figure 7.1 are included in the following box.

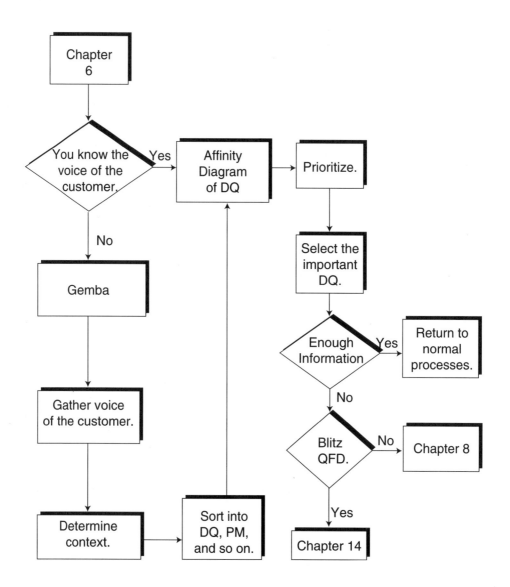

If this is a learning exercise, sketch a high-level process map of how your service fits into your customer's process or life.

If this is an actual QFD project, ask your customer to describe their process.

THE VOICE-OF-THE-CUSTOMER TABLE, PART 1

When the QFD team went into the Gemba, they recorded what the customers had to say in a *voice-of-the-customer table, part 1 (VOCT1)*. A *5W1H format* (who, what, when, where, why, and how), as modified by Mazur (1996), is shown in Figure 7.2.

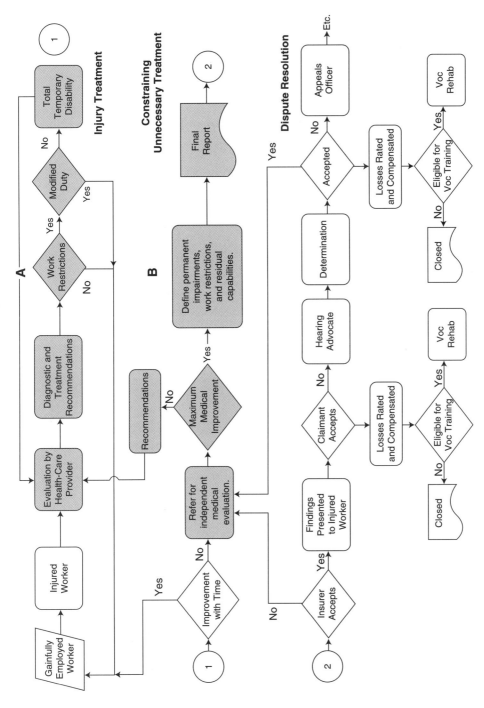

Figure 7.1. High-level view of customer's process. The first row focuses on treating the acute injuries. The second row shows activities that constrain unnecessary treatment. A series of activities and tasks in the third row outlines activities for the dispute resolution. The organization in the case example provided tasks and functions shaded in the second row, labeled B.

Figure 7.1 Process Details

Workers' compensation insurance plans are designed to provide medical treatment of insured workers, temporary replacement of wages while recovering if they are not able to work, and compensation for lost work capacity if they experience a loss in function that is a permanent loss. The portion of the workers' compensation system pertinent to this project is sketched as a flowchart in the figure. The first row of functions is for treating injuries; the second is for constraining unnecessary care; and the third is for dispute resolution.

Most workers who receive treatment and temporary disability payments improve and return to being gainfully employed. Some, however, continue a cycle of reevaluations, recommendations, treatment, continued total temporary disability, reevaluation, and so on (shaded blocks *A,* Figure 7.1). In part of row two, in some of these cases, the intensity of symptoms and/or the claimed physical impairments persist beyond what the usual recovery time is for such an injury and/or the symptoms and claimed impairments seem to be far out of proportion to the degree of injury. If this apparent state persists for an inordinately long period of time, insurers may refer the injured workers for an independent medical evaluation (IME). Since many such workers have complex injuries involving multiple parts of the body or organ systems, such an evaluation frequently involves multiple specialists and diagnostic studies.

As part of an IME, a determination is made as to whether this person has experienced maximal medical improvement or not. If not, appropriate recommendations are made and carried out by a treating healthcare provider. If maximum medical improvement has occurred, by definition no further diagnostic or medical treatments have a reasonable probability of reducing symptoms, improving function, or increasing employability. In those cases, the independent medical evaluators also define permanent impairments, permanent work restrictions, and residual functional capacities. The medical record, shown as a final report, becomes a record of these findings.

Upon receipt of the report(s), the insurer may be satisfied or dissatisfied with the result. If the insurer does not accept the findings, because they either are incomplete or do not seem appropriate, further independent medical evaluation may be requested. If the insurer does accept the findings, these findings are presented to the injured worker. If the worker accepts these findings and has significant loss in physical capacity and employability, the losses are rated and compensation for the losses is determined. If the worker cannot return to his or her previous job or organization, he or she may be qualified for vocational rehabilitation. Vocational rehabilitation evaluation is obtained, and recommendations are made and followed. The degree of impairment is rated by a qualified "rating physician," and compensation for permanent losses in function is determined.

If the worker does not accept the findings of the IME, the worker—and most workers at this point usually have an attorney—requests an administrative hearing. The hearing officer may determine that further independent medical evaluation or further treatment is indicated or no further evaluations are indicated. If the recommendation of the hearing officer is further medical evaluation and this is accepted by the insurer and the worker, that is carried out. If both the insurer and the injured worker accept a hearing determination that no further evaluation is indicated, impairments are rated and a determination is made whether the worker is eligible for vocational rehabilitation. If either the insurer or the worker does not accept the determination of the hearing officer, a hearing by an appeals officer can be initiated, and so on.

The customer's response was recorded verbatim in column 1. Then the who, what, when, where, why, and how that build a context for that response were entered in the next columns. Exact words are recorded, not the team's interpretation or potential solution. It is also important to include any information about the customer that would influence the service or how the customer might use the service. This sounds simple but in practice may not be. Provider biases and paternalistic tendencies, like the Ames's room, can shape what is heard and affect provider responses. The following questions will help guide the team in the collection of useful customer information.

The Who?

- Who uses the service?

- Who else may use the service?

- Who may use the service in the future?

- Keep asking the question, "Who is missing?"

The What?

- What are the services used for?

- What else might the services be used for both now and in the future?

- What future uses do you see for the service?

- Keep asking the question, "What is missing?"

The primary use for your service in the customer's environment may be different for different people within that environment. For example, for the nurse case manager, the service's primary benefit was to determine if further treatment was necessary. For the claims examiner, it often was expense control. For personnel in the legal department, it was dispute resolution. Similarly, the role of a service in a geriatric population may be viewed one way by the geriatric patient and another way by the family and the community.

The Where?

- Where is the service used?

- Where else might the service be used now and in the future?

- Keep asking the question, "What variation of *where* is missing?"

Cust Info	Voice of the Customer	Who, What, When, Where	Why	How	Reworded Data
	We want to know if drugs are involved.	Who: Nurse Case Manager What: Street Drugs When: Inpatient Evaluations Where: In Injured Worker	Find Illicit Drugs	Blood and Urine	We need screening for drugs.
	Except for name at the top, all the reports from some evaluation centers look and say the same thing.	Who: Legal Advocate What: Final Reports When: At Appeals Where: At Appeals	Credibility at Appeals	Individualized and Specific Case Reports	Individualized case-specific reports are created.
	Medical facts speak louder than medical opinions.	Who: Claims Examiner What: Distinguishing Criteria When: When Findings Contested Where: Negotiations or Appeals	Weight When Conflicting Opinions	Opinions Grounded by facts and Observations	Opinions are linked to facts wherever possible.
	Psychiatric impairments are barriers to vocational rehab.	Who: Nurse Case Manager What: Psychiatric Problems When: Getting Back to Work Where: In Vocational Retraining	Are Barriers to Return to Work	Motivation Reduced by Anxiety and Depression	Psychiatric issues can be barriers to return to work.
	Psychiatric problems are covered only if there was extreme danger at time of injury (i.e., victim of violent crimes).	Who: RN What: Psychiatric Problems When: Recommendations Where: Treatment	Reduce Frivolous Stress Claims	By Regulation	Only rarely is psychiatric treatment a covered benefit.

Figure 7.2. Sample voice-of-the-customer table, Part 1 (VOCT1). The voice of the customer is captured by interviewing customers in the field, and the data is entered into the table.

Many hospital services are used within the hospital itself. Though being used within the hospital, a service may influence customer's behavior, wants, and needs in locations outside the hospital. For example, a person who falls and fractures a hip has the hip repaired and undergoes rehabilitation to walk in a facility. But they will return to walk in an environment, such as the home, which may be filled with hazards to safe walking.

The When?

- When is the service used?

- When may the service be used now and in the future?

- Keep asking the question, "What variation of *when* is missing?"

In the case study, the service was currently used after all alternatives for such a complex evaluation were explored. Is it possible that using the service earlier would reduce overall costs and improve outcomes?

The Why?

- Why is the service now used?

- Why might it be used?

- Keep asking the question, "Why is this service used instead of some alternative?"

- Identify alternatives that are used. Why are they used?

Why a service is used is not the same as what it is used for. In our example, *what* the service is used for is outlined in the customer's process chart (Figure 7.1). However, *why* the customer chooses to use the service now as opposed to earlier or later and *why* they choose one particular service over another can be very different.

The customer's first response to the question "Why?" may not uncover the true need. Often, asking a *why* question several times uncovers more fundamental needs. Asking "Why is that important?" or "Why do you need that?" are variations of the five whys of the Toyota production process (Ohno 1988).

The How?

- How is the service used?

- How else might the service be used now and in the future?

Reworded Data: Expanding the Verbatim Response

In this section, the customer's voice is expanded and integrated to generate more detailed data. For example, in the VOCT1 (Figure 7.2) the verbatim response from the customer was, "Except for the name, the reports from some places are the same." This comment came from a person in the legal department who felt such reports lacked credibility. This was reworded to customer wants "individualized case-specific reports." If any of the customer verbatim statements contain more than one idea, they must be separated into individual statements. Statements are reworded as positive statements for ease of analysis in setting targets later.

EXERCISE 7.2

If this is a practice workshop, generate a list of 20 customer statements and enter these into the first column of the VOCT1 (blank sample in Appendix A). If this is an actual project, interview actual customer segments selected in chapter 6 at the location where your service is used.

EXERCISE 7.3

Complete who, what, when, where, why, and how.

This is another opportunity to identify what may be missing. The context of 5W1H identifies customer needs. Linking novel combinations of the 5W and 1H may identify additional needs. Combining the 5W and 1H with the verbatim data identifies additional needs. Customers do not say everything that is important to them. This is one way to create a more complete set of customer demands.

EXERCISE 7.4

Expand the verbatim response by rewording and integrating the data with 5W1H.

Suggestions and Cautions

What is the optimal number of customers to interview in the field? Organizations need to observe and interview only 15 to 20 customers in depth. Research shows that the added benefits of interviewing or observing more than 20 customers are marginal. However, this suggested sample size of 15 to 20 is for *each* customer segment of interest. If you are going to design your services for three customer segments, 45 people (15 from each segment) would need to be interviewed.

With provider biases and paternalistic tendencies, some interviewers experience disbelief or denial about what the customer is saying, "How could he/she want that?" "That doesn't make any sense." Remember, the goal in capturing the voice of the customer is to do just that, capture the actual stimuli presented to you by the customer. The who, what, when, where, why, and how components of the table are used to expand your understanding of what the customer means by his or her statement and, if possible, actually witness how the service is used.

THE VOICE-OF-THE-CUSTOMER TABLE, PART 2

Entries in the voice-of-the-customer and reworded data columns from VOCT1 usually contain a heterogeneous mixture of statements about the service. For example, the columns will probably contain not only demanded qualities but also statements about performance, failures, functions, and price. The following definitions will be used to characterize voice-of-the-customer data:

Demanded Quality

- Answers the question, "What performance does your customer want?" Often found by asking why the customer wants "X."

- What is driving the demanded quality? This is revealed by continually asking "Why?" to the answer just given. Ask "Why?" five times or until you appear to be frustrating the customer. Be creative by asking "Why?" without using the word "why" in the question.

- A demanded quality is usually expressed as an adverb and as a verb but is sometimes stated as a verb, adjective, and object.

- For ease of subsequent analysis, demanded qualities are expressed by positive statements.

  Example: The customer says "I want to be evaluated quickly." The demanded quality is quick evaluation.

Performance Measures (Sometimes Called Quality Characteristics or Quality Attributes)

- Measures the quality of a function and includes units of measure. Initially it is not necessary to know how to accomplish the measuring, only what is to be measured. Major breakthroughs in technologies and processes occur with the advent of new measurement systems. Before a comparison between the existing, alternative, and competing systems is possible, a means of measure must be identified or created. The measurement must be an effective predictor of customer satisfaction, or it is not useful.

  Example: The time requirement to evaluate the patient is identified as the Performance Measure. The zero point is when the organization is first aware of the patient, and the duration ends when the final report is delivered to the appropriate people. There are many other intervals that could be called the "time to evaluate." This one would be selected because it includes all of the time during which the organization could be doing something or has a responsibility to begin. It is the cycle time for the service.

Function

- What does the service do?

- What tasks are performed?

- Function is expressed as a noun, an active verb, and an object.

Failure Mode

- Expressed as a deficit. Typically a negative statement.

  Example: "The age is wrong in the report."

Each of these is used at a different step in the QFD process. Correctly separating the data by these categories is important to building a robust and effective QFD system.

All items are entered into the VOCT2. Any item that is not a demanded quality should be represented by a corresponding demanded quality that is also added to the demanded quality list. For example, in Figure 7.3, the common failure noted as *Recommend psychiatric or psychological treatment for noncovered conditions* is listed as a breakdown or failure in current services. The demanded quality might be rephrased as *Recommend psychiatric or psychological treatment only for covered services.* This is yet another chance to identify what may be missing. Again, demanded qualities are listed as positive statements.

Cust ID	Demanded Quality	Performance Measures	Function	Reliability	Failure Modes	Other
RN		Reports of Drug Screen				
Legal	Individualized and Case-Specific Reports					
CE		Opinion Linked to Facts				
CE				Identify psychiatric problems that could be barriers to retraining and work.		
RN					Recommend psychiatric or psychological treatments for noncovered conditions.	

Figure 7.3. Sample voice-of-the customer table, Part 2 (VOCT2). Data from the VOCT1 is separated into demanded qualities, performance measures, functions, reliability, and failure mode.

The readers may find they disagree with some of the reworded data or sorting of data in the case study. However, to fully appreciate how the particular items in the tables were agreed upon, one would have had to participate in the discussions.

Sometimes the demanded qualities or reworded data are long, and teams use one-to-two-word phrases to characterize them. If this is done, it is very important to have a glossary defining the abbreviations attached to the original statement or the reworded data. An example of a glossary is shown in Appendix B. We tend to interpret stimuli through the background or context within which the stimuli were presented to us. The Ames's room (Figure 2.3) demonstrates this visually. As the teams move through the QFD process, a term may provoke one set of assessments in, for example, VOCT and another set of assessments under function deployment. When this happens, the team loses sight of the target. The measure, function, and linkage from customer to task can break down. Similarly, if there is any discussion about the significance of a particular voiced statement or reworded data, a discussion about its interpretation should occur and agreement as to interpretation should be recorded in the glossary.

The glossary becomes very important in function and task-deployment phases. It is here that the team begins to confront how they or their department will have to change their behaviors to achieve the agreed-upon targets. It is here that the existing homeostatic feedback in the *as is* systems of the organization (whether formal, informal, individual, or collective) begins to reexert itself, consciously or unconsciously. The organization will try to return to the safety of the known, to slide from Point 2 back to Point 1 on the archetypal map of change (Figure 2.9). This tendency may appear as questioning of what is really important. The team may face what appears to be a difficult or impossible task of measuring, collecting selected performance measures, reaching improvement targets, and so on. Do not be discouraged. In every redesign project, there this is already an *as is* system in place, with both operational and political dimensions. This existing system contains historical targets and hemostatic feedback loops that self-organize the space and maintain the status quo of the organization.

EXERCISE 7.5

Complete VOCT2 by rewording the data from VOCT1, and sort the statements as demanded qualities, performance measures, functions, and failure modes (blank form in Appendix A).

EXERCISE 7.6

Identify all the missing demanded qualities that relate to the non–demanded quality statements in the VOCT2.

SORTING AND GROUPING DATA

Affinity Diagram: Sorting Demanded Qualities into Natural Clusters or Groups

All demanded qualities are recorded on 3 × 5 index cards or large Post-it® Notes. The letters on the cards or Post-its® should be large enough for the people sorting them to read at a distance of one yard. A group of customers (if this is a practice exercise, team members) are assembled. In the case study, nine customers (including claims examiners, RN case managers, and members of the legal department) were assembled and 3×5 cards were used.

The cards are placed on a table in random order. Post-it® Notes can be positioned on a vertical surface, again, in random order. Some walls have a coating to reduce dust collection and to enhance cleaning. Repositionable notes only stay on this surface for 15 minutes. You might want to test your wall.

If the people doing the sorting have not seen the complete list, take a moment to read all the demanded qualities. The group then gathers around the wall or table and quickly, without talking (silently), organizes the notes into related groups. In our example, the customers were asked to form groups of no more than four demanded qualities. If one of the sorters finds a demanded quality is not where they think it should be, he or she moves it to another group. The process continues until all demanded qualities are grouped. If one demanded quality is moved multiple times between groups, consider making a duplicate of that quality and placing it with both groups. Sometimes a "group" may contain only one demanded quality. These single-item groups may not represent a true demanded quality and may require special treatment during the design phase.

The construction of an affinity diagram is touted to be a right-brain activity. The process is similar to giving children several shapes and asking them to group them by asking the questions, "How are these things the same?" or "How are they alike?" Many practitioners recommend that the nondominant hand be used for repositioning items during the affinity process.

After the grouping activity seems to have become somewhat stable, review with the customers (team members) doing the sorting those demanded qualities that seem to have more than one home. This may bring out different interpretations of the demanded quality's meaning.

Next, a descriptive title or name is selected for each group. These group names should also be phrased as demanded qualities (adverb and verb; or sometimes verb, adjective, and object). These groupings are also demanded qualities but at a higher level of abstraction. Figure 7.4 presents a sample for two named clusters from the case example. It is useful to look at the group names and ask the question, "In this group name, what elements should be included but are missing?" This question uncovers additional and sometimes important demanded qualities.

Next, the groupings are challenged by asking the question, "When considering all aspects of this service, are any aspects not represented by the group headings?" Again, this is to see if any important qualities are missing. When the affinity diagram was first done in our example, *More help in managing local MDs* was not there but was added after asking the question of what was missing. If the first grouping generates more than nine group headings, the groupings are again grouped according to the affinity process. In the case example, data was grouped into three levels of abstraction. One level was verbatim or reworded data captured in the field. The next two levels were abstracted data from the affinity process.

An affinity diagram is a tool to sort and provide structure to verbal data, in this case the demanded qualities, by creating clusters or groups of related items. The output presents a visual format or map of the data in much the same way that a scatter diagram might be used to enhance the interpretation and assessments of raw nominal data.

Both the affinity diagram and tree hierarchy (discussed next) are used to ensure that the list of demanded qualities is complete. Both tools also help verify that all of the group headings are at the same level of abstraction and all of the elements in a group

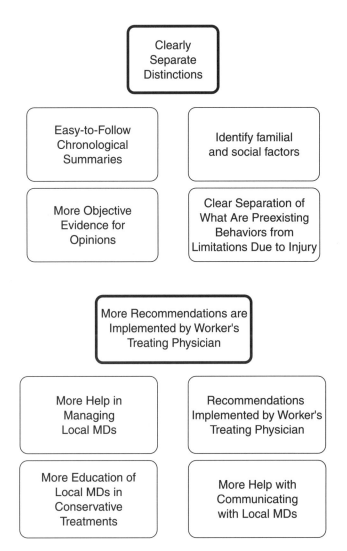

Figure 7.4. Affinity diagram for demanded qualities. Two sample groupings from the total affinity diagram of demanded quality statements are shown. "More help in managing local MDs" was added after the groups were formed.

are at the same level of abstraction. The same level of abstraction is needed for using the AHP process and for designing a questionnaire, which will be needed later.

SUGGESTIONS AND CAUTIONS

1. Optimal number of people to do the sorting is 7 + or − 2.

2. If there are more elements in one group than in the other groups, this may mean that it is really two or more groups. It is best to divide any group with more than five items, just to make sure.

3. If there are more than 9 groups after the first round of sorting, the groups themselves must be grouped.

Summary for Construction of Affinity Diagram

- All Demanded Qualities are placed on 3 × 5 cards or Post-it® Notes and placed randomly on a table or wall.
- A representative group gathers around the flat surface (a table or wall) where demanded qualities have been randomly placed.
- Everyone participates.
- The group *silently* organizes the demanded qualities into related groupings. This is done quickly, with no analysis.
- The group keeps placing and moving the demanded qualities (making duplicates when needed) until some stability is reached.
- Working in silence helps to balance strong and mild personalities. Right-handed people should use their left hand to move cards around, and left-handed people should use their right hand.
- When groupings are stable, label each group by its theme or affinity (a demanded quality at a higher level of abstraction) with a different colored card or Post-it® Note. These group headings may then be grouped again, until two or three levels have been identified.
- Missing groups and missing elements of groups are added.

---

4. Single items may not be demanded qualities, or they may be so unique in nature that they will require special treatment during the design process.

5. When developing names for affinity group categories, avoid generic and vague modifiers such as "good."

6. When selecting descriptive names for groups of demanded qualities, take advantage of new insights and avoid a dominant participant trying to talk everyone into using some traditional grouping.

7. When groupings in the affinity process are customer driven, the natural clusters for demanded qualities that are formed often provide more insight than any structured questionnaire or focus group would.

EXERCISE 7.7

Make 3 × 5 cards or large Post-it® Notes for your demanded qualities. If this is a practice or learning exercise, the team sorts the data. If this is an actual project, a group of customers sorts the data.

- Data is placed randomly on a table or wall.
- Group the notes quickly without talking, and use the nondominant hand.
- When the process appears to be stabilized, stop the sorting.
- Name groupings as demanded qualities.
- Sort the named groups, and name the grouped groupings.
- Question: Are all of the elements of the group at the same level of abstraction? If one of the elements is more general, can it be used as a group name?
- Are there any missing groups? Add these.
- Are there any missing elements in any of the groups? Add these.
- The data are now ready to be placed in a tree diagram.

Tree Diagram for Prioritizing Demanded Qualities

The *tree diagram* provides a method to ensure that levels of abstraction are symmetrical and to identify potentially missing demanded qualities. A tree can be constructed in one of two ways: from the branches toward the trunk, or from the trunk toward the branches.

When the results of an affinity diagram are used, the tree starts with the leaves and works toward the trunk. In the case study, the demanded qualities from the voice-of-the-customer and reworded data were the leaves and the two levels of the affinity process provided the branches and trunk.

Look at each level to see if there is anything missing at that level. Is there something in the level that is more global or finer detail than the rest of the demanded qualities in that level? Make the necessary adjustment by moving the entry and all of its component details to the appropriate level.

A segment of the tree diagram from the case example is shown in Figure 7.5. In Figures 7.5 and 7.6, high-level (Level A) entries are shown with AHP ratings, but lower levels of the tree (Levels B and C) are only shown for *Improved physician communication*. There were seven groupings at this level (only three are shown in Level A, in the Figures).

After the tree diagram is constructed, the demanded qualities in the tree are ranked or prioritized. This can be accomplished in two ways. One method uses AHP, and the other uses the distribution of 100 points. The team in our example used AHP to weight the elements of the tree. The AHP process began with the level (A) of abstraction, which included *Improved physician communication* (Figure 7.6). These items were entered into the rows and columns of an AHP table similar to that shown in chapter 6. The same group of customers who constructed the affinity diagram then did pairwise comparisons using the nine-point scale. The final results were expressed as a percentage, as noted in Figure 7.6. *Improved physician communication* was ranked as 22.14 percent.

The team then set up a table for pairwise comparisons for the next level (Level B in Figure 7.6). Using the pairwise comparison method (AHP), the subgroups for *Improved physician communication* were compared and weights were found to be 16.6 percent for *Better MD communication of findings to injured workers* and 83.4 percent for *More MD follow-through in implementing recommendations* (shown as a percent, not bold, in the tree). These weights need to be adjusted for the weight of the higher category of which they are parts. Therefore, the weight, expressed as a fraction for each of these two items, is multiplied by the weight as a percent of its group heading. For example, *Better MD communication of findings to injured workers* is 16% of the weight of its higher grouping, so 0.166×22.14, yields 3.67. This is shown in bold in the tree diagram above the percentage. These values are then related to the value or weight of the higher group so that, when the tree is complete, the different branches (e.g., Level B) can be directly compared to each other.

Similarly, the next level, which in this tree would be the leaves (Labeled C), is weighted using the AHP process. The weights obtained are then multiplied by the weight for the higher level to determine the weight for each item at this level. Again, during the AHP process it is important to make your comparisons at the same level of abstraction. In this way, the weights are carried throughout the entire tree. Any elements within Level A can be compared with all elements at Level A, and all elements in Level B can be compared with all other elements at Level B, and so on.

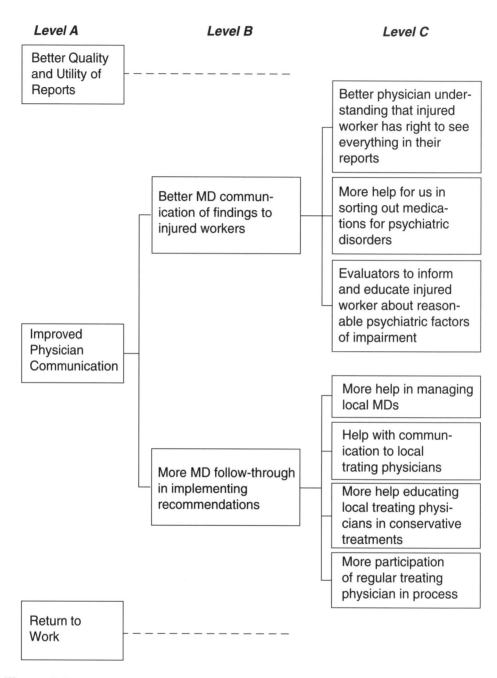

Figure 7.5. Affinity diagram as a tree. The affinity diagram was converted to a tree structure for ranking. Only one branch of the tree is shown in detail. The complete tree is in Appendix E.

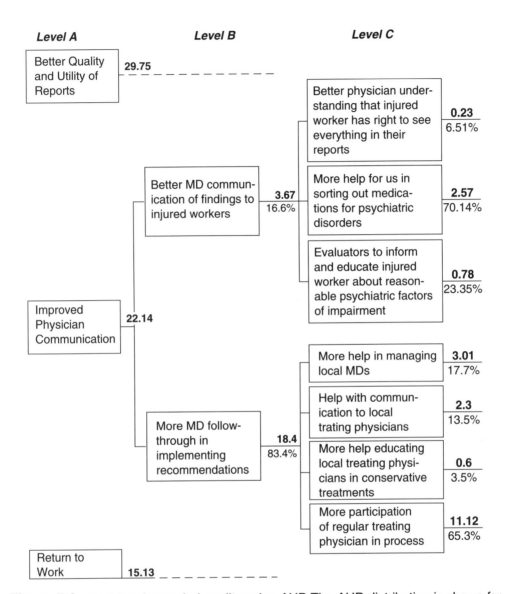

Figure 7.6. Ranking demanded quality using AHP. The AHP distribution is shown for one branch. The bold number at the top is the relative importance as distributed by the percentage shown.

Another method for prioritizing demanded qualities within the tree is the distribution of 100 points. Here, 100 points are distributed among the group headings, such as at Level A. If 20 points were allocated to *Improved physician communication,* then these 20 points would next be allocated between *Better MD communication of findings to injured workers* and *More MD follow-through in implementing recommendations.*

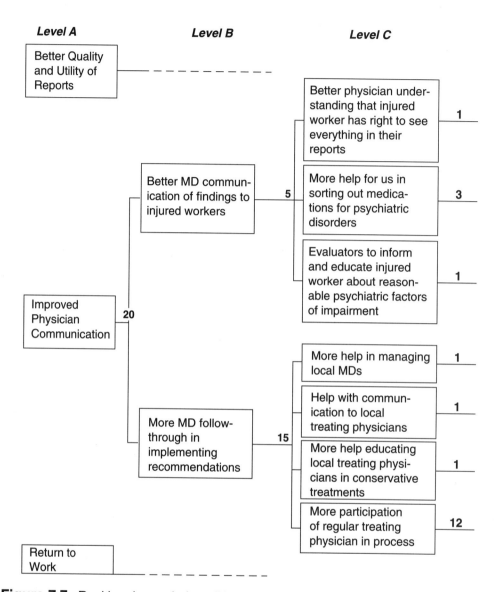

Figure 7.7. Ranking demanded qualities using 100 points. An alternative for ranking but not recommended is distributing 100 points from the trunk of the tree to the smallest branch.

Similarly, the distribution of points is worked out to the next lower level (Figure 7.7). Upon completing the Affinity Diagram, the Tree and AHP Process, or Distribution of 100 Points to weight demanded qualities on the tree, the team in the case example selected the eight items that ranked highest in this process. These items were used to design a customer survey.

SUGGESTIONS AND CAUTIONS

According to Saaty, the maximum number of branches for any level of comparison is nine. If you have more than nine branches, the data need to be broken down into sub-groupings. Before grouping, make sure there are not repeat entries.

Prioritization of demanded qualities should come from a group of customers and not from the QFD team. When the QFD team carries out this step, preconceived biases and paternalistic tendencies are reintroduced into the process.

AHP takes time and can try the customer's patience. As a market becomes more mature or competitive, however, companies move from simple, ordinal data to the use of AHP. This information is invaluable to the provider since this process allows sensitive items to rise to top priority.

In one QFD project, the goal was to improve the internal performance of the hospital. The highest-ranked demanded quality was *Improved capacity to keep commitments,* meaning a major problem for the organization, including the QFD team, was in keeping commitments they had made. When this was initially included as one of a list of possible areas for improvement, there was much heated discussion. Several team members argued that meeting commitments was not really a problem. After ranking 42 items for improvement through AHP, this demanded quality was evaluated as the highest. With this support, there was little resistance to its importance.

EXERCISE 7.8

- Place the affinity groupings from Exercise 7.7 into a tree.
- Is the tree balanced? If not, take corrective action.
- Prioritize the demanded qualities within the tree by using AHP or distribution of 100 points.

DESIGNING A QUESTIONNAIRE

The team in our example selected demanded qualities from Level B of abstraction. This kept the effort for the team and the customer modest and useful—sometimes less is more. For example, using Level C in the questionnaire was possible, but then customers might have had to use the 100 points for many of the 61 leaves (Level C). The number of demanded qualities also influences the level of detail in the QFD process. The heart of the QFD process is the *matrix tool.* It will require time to evaluate all the cells in the matrix. The number of cells is equal to the product of the rows and columns, so the number of demanded qualities selected to carry throughout the process will determine the size of the matrix. If the team had chosen all 61 demanded qualities identified in the field for the questionnaire, at least 3721 relationships would need to be evaluated in the matrix table and during later steps. The number of items that was selected for the questionnaire and then the number of items to be selected to enter into the Quality Planning Table, therefore, set a context for the level of detail that will be carried throughout the QFD process. The eight selected Demanded Qualities were:

1. More comprehensive evaluations

2. More comprehensive reports

3. Definition of all findings as pre- or postinjury

4. Better work capacity assessments

5. More treating physician follow-through with recommendations

6. More acceptance of findings at appeal hearings

7. Independence from insurers maintained

8. More understandable reports

The nature of the data captured using the tools described came from selected customers and is qualitative in nature. This data is used to design a survey to collect information from a larger sample of the customer population. Data from such surveys is more quantitative in nature.

The questionnaire for the case study will be used as an example. The questionnaire had three parts. Part 1 used a five-point scale (1 for "does not matter" to 5 for "very strongly matters") to rate the eight demanded qualities selected from the tree diagram. The eight selected demanded qualities were included in the full questionnaire. Part 1 of the questionnaire tests whether qualitative data captured in the field is quantitatively important for a larger sample of the population of customers (Figure 7.8).

Part 2 of the questionnaire also used a five-point scale (1 for "poor" to 5 for "excellent") to compare the services of the rehabilitation hospital to three of its competitors. Part 2 of the questionnaire competitively ranked the organization and its competitors on each of the eight selected items (Figure 7.9). Part 3 of the questionnaire asked pairs of multiple-choice questions. The first half of the pair asks how customers would feel if an item was present. The second half asks how they would feel if it was not present. These paired questions are tools used for the Kano Model for understanding the importance of various features of a service. Features in this model are called *needs*. The paired questions describe the level of performance for the demanded qualities (Figure 7.10). One question is in the form, "How would you feel if XX was provided?" The second question is in the form, "How would you feel if XX was not provided?" The possible answers are:

1   I like it that way.
2   I expect it.
3   I feel neutral.
4   I can tolerate it.
5   I dislike it that way.

Customer responses to direct questions about what quality they expect are often fuzzy and difficult to interpret. However, their responses tend to fall into three types of assessments: basic needs, performance needs, and excitement needs. For some customer requirements, customer satisfaction is proportional to how fully functional the product or service is. These are performance needs as shown in Figure 7.11. The vertical axis represents the customer's level of satisfaction, and the horizontal axis represents the level of quality for a function. For performance needs, the customer is more satisfied when performance is better. Performance needs are shown as a solid line in the figure.

For other requirements, the need is so fundamental that it may not even be verbalized by the customer. These are basic needs. The best performance for a basic need will only result in a customer who is not unhappy. That is, the customer is unhappy if the need is unsatisfied but is not more satisfied if the need's function is improved. You would be unhappy if the tire on the airplane in which you were landing blew out and made for

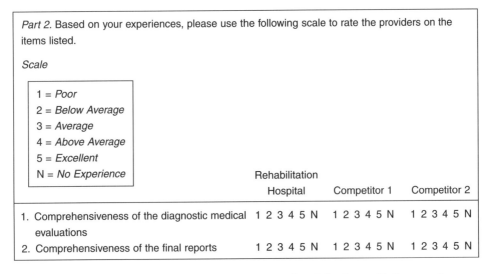

Part 1. Using a scale where *1 = Does Not Matter* and *5 = Very Strongly Matters,* please rate how the following factors influence your decisions when deciding on whom to make a referral to for complex independent evaluations for injured workers.

	Does Not Matter	Somewhat Matters	Matters	Strongly Matters	Very Strongly Matters
1. Previous experience with the comprehensiveness of diagnostic medical evaluations	1	2	3	4	5
2. Previous experience with comprehensiveness of final reports	1	2	3	4	5

Figure 7.8. Questionnaire, Part 1. The customers' importance for the demanded qualities is found using a Likert scale.

Part 2. Based on your experiences, please use the following scale to rate the providers on the items listed.

Scale

1 = *Poor*
2 = *Below Average*
3 = *Average*
4 = *Above Average*
5 = *Excellent*
N = *No Experience*

	Rehabilitation Hospital	Competitor 1	Competitor 2
1. Comprehensiveness of the diagnostic medical evaluations	1 2 3 4 5 N	1 2 3 4 5 N	1 2 3 4 5 N
2. Comprehensiveness of the final reports	1 2 3 4 5 N	1 2 3 4 5 N	1 2 3 4 5 N

Figure 7.9. Questionnaire, Part 2. The customers' satisfaction with the services provided for the demanded qualities is found using a Likert scale.

rough landing, but you are not excited by the service of an airline just because the plane lands smoothly. Improving on basic needs will not enhance customer satisfaction. It is a waste of resources that can be used to improve a performance need or introduce an excitement need. Basic needs fall below the lower dotted line in Figure 7.11.

Often, excitement needs are also not verbalized. Excitement needs, however, provide the opportunity of creating immediate customer happiness and enthusiasm. Excitement needs fall above the upper dotted line on the Kano Model.

In practice, a table is usually used to interpret the results of Part 3 of the questionnaire (Figure 7.12). There are 25 possible combinations for the paired questions. Their interpretation is shown in the figure. The answers to negatively phrased questions

Part 3. This last section asks pairs of multiple-choice questions. Half of the questions ask how you would feel if an item was present; the other half asks how you would feel if the item was not present. Simply select the answer that seems most appropriate for you.

1a. If the diagnostic medical evaluation appears comprehensive, how do you feel?

   5. I like it that way.
   4. It must be that way.
   3. I am neutral.
   2. I can live with it that way.
   1. I dislike it that way.

1b. If the diagnostic medical evaluation does not seem comprehensive, how do you feel?

   5. I like it that way.
   4. It must be that way.
   3. I am neutral.
   2. I can live with it that way.
   1. I dislike it that way.

Figure 7.10. Questionnaire, Part 3. Paired questions are used to determine the type of need of the demanded qualities. The questions are phrased as a function being provided and not provided.

identify the column. The answers to the positively phrased questions identify the row. The cells with the *Q* indicate that the response was inconsistent. The cells with the *I* indicate an indifferent response.

The cells with the *RB, RP,* and *RE* indicate a reverse response for Basic Need, Performance Need, and Exciting Need. A reverse response occurs when the respondent dislikes the positive and likes the negative. If both normal and reverse responses occur in the raw data, there are two customer segments. This might happen if both a smoker and a nonsmoker are asked, "How would you feel if smoking was allowed?" and "How would you feel if smoking was not allowed?" In contrast to a nonsmoker, a smoker in California would probably have a pair of answers rated as excitement (Row 5, Column 4). They would be excited if they were allowed to smoke in a restaurant since smoking is not permitted.

The raw data for the demanded quality *More comprehensive evaluations* is shown in Figure 7.13. We see that most of the responses (19) were in cell (4,1), which is a basic response.

The data from Part 3 of the case study questionnaire can be recorded as shown in Figure 7.14. We see that Demanded Qualities *2, 3, 4,* and *6* are performance needs, *5* and *8* are excitement needs, and *1* is a basic need: *7* is an indifferent response. This would suggest that *G* is not very important.

EXERCISE 7.9

- Select three demanded qualities.
- Create the paired questions for each demanded quality.
- Have the team members record their answers.
- What distribution of results do you have? How many basic, performance, or excitement needs are there?

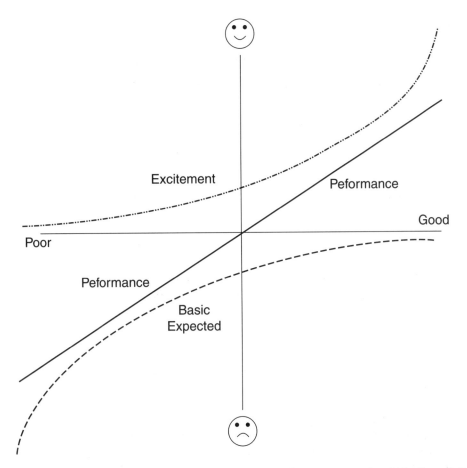

Figure 7.11. Kano Model. The Kano Model shows the customers' satisfaction plotted against a function performance. Exciting functions are viewed positively by just being offered. Performance functions are more positive if viewed as providing better performance. Basic functions are expected, and the best that can be expected by the customer is a neutral feeling.

EXERCISE 7.10

Prepare a questionnaire:
- Design a questionnaire that ranks the demanded qualities from Exercise 7.8 on a five-point scale (1 for "does not matter" to 5 for "very strongly matters"), as shown in Figure 7.8.
- Identify competitive rankings for current service providers based on your experience. Use a five-point scale to rate how you and other   providers do on delivering demanded qualities (1 for "poor" to 5 for "excellent").
- Design a competitive rating questionaire as shown in Figure 7.9.
- Design a series of prepared questions for a Kano analysis of the demanded qualities used in Exercise 7.10.

			How do you feel if XX is not provided?				
			5	4	3	2	1
			I like it.	I expect it.	I feel neutral.	I can tolerate it.	I dislike it.
Functional	5	I like it.	Q	E	E	E	P
	4	I expect it.	RE	Q	I	I	B
How do you feel if XX is provided?	3	I feel neutral.	RE	I	I	I	B
	2	I can tolerate it.	RE	I	I	Q	B
	1	I dislike it.	RP	RB	RB	RB	Q

Requirement is

E: Exciting   P: Performance
B: Basic   Q: Questionable
R: Reverse   I: Indifferent

Figure 7.12. Kano types. The 25 different responses for the paired Kano questions are shown. Each is assigned an interpretation of Basic, Performance, or Exciting.

			How do you feel if XX is not provided?				
			5	4	3	2	1
			I like it.	I expect it.	I feel neutral.	I can tolerate it.	I dislike it.
Functional	5	I like it.					9
	4	I expect it.					19
How do you feel if XX is provided?	3	I feel neutral.					3
	2	I can tolerate it.					1
	1	I dislike it.					

Figure 7.13. Kano raw data. The response frequencies for the paired questions associated with the demanded quality *Diagnostic medical evaluations are comprehensive and complete* are recorded.

SUGGESTIONS AND CAUTIONS

How many demanded qualities should an organization select? The answer is, it depends in part on the complexity of the service, the maturity and complexity of the market within which the service competes, and the level of sophistication of the organization. If this is your first QFD project, smaller is probably better. Selecting too general a level of abstraction carries the risk of producing a very small matrix of limited

			How do you feel if XX is not provided?				
			5	4	3	2	1
			I like it.	I expect it.	I feel neutral.	I can tolerate it.	I dislike it.
Functional	5	I like it.			5	8	2,3,4,6
	4	I expect it.					1
How do you feel if XX is provided?	3	I feel neutral.					
	2	I can tolerate it.			7		
	1	I dislike it.					

Summary of Results
Exciting   5,8
Performance   2,3,4,6
Basic   1
Indifferent   7

Figure 7.14. Kano data for all demanded qualities. The location for each demanded quality is shown for the Kano Model.

value. Selecting a very large number causes complexities in the evaluative process that can sink the project. As a rule of thumb, 20 to 30 demanded qualities are comfortable to analyze and provide useful insight for an experienced team. The team in our example chose eight, in part because this was their first project and in part because it was their assessment that improving these eight demanded qualities would achieve their goals of increasing referrals to the service. The team might have chosen to design a questionnaire based on the Kano model and to collect sample data for this part of their questionnaire before sending the questionnaire to a larger sample of the customer population. This strategy would have allowed the team to build a more refined questionnaire for ranking the demanded qualities and the competitive analysis. For example, the item *Independence from insurers maintained* would have been noted to be in a different range and probably not included in the questionnaire designed to generate more quantitative data. If the team had used 30 demanded qualities in their questionnaire, this would have generated the need for 120 responses from the customers—30 ranking importance rating, 30 for competitive ranking, and 60 for the Kano Analysis. Their assessment was that this number of responses would markedly reduce the number of returned questionnaires.

As a product/service improves, the customer's perceived needs become more demanding. What was an excitement need yesterday becomes a performance need today and a basic need tomorrow. Likewise, at times, a dramatic improvement in performance can generate excitement, or a new technology for the basic need sets a new standard for performance.

Consider X rays and X-ray reports. Initially X rays were taken and interpreted by the ordering physician. The physician as a customer was satisfied by a good quality X ray. Later, radiology developed as a physician specialty. As a customer, the ordering physician might be satisfied if he or she gets a report from the radiologist in the mail and can go look at any abnormal X rays he or she wishes to see. When faxes became available, getting a report faxed to the ordering physician the same day generated excitement. Today, this is the expected level of performance. Now, the ability to log onto an intranet and to both see the X ray and simultaneously read or hear the radiologist's report is what generates excitement.

Features that excite customers today will become expected features or qualities tomorrow. In order to ensure competitive services in a rapidly changing environment, organizations must keep in touch with their customers so that they know when their customers' needs are changing. The organization must also keep in touch with emerging technologies that are disruptive because they do not fit into the current pattern.

SUGGESTIONS AND CAUTIONS

Affinity diagrams, the tree structure, and AHP begin to answer the question, "What is important to the customer?" These results may not meet either the organization's nor the team members' initial expectations. As data is collected, weighted, and ranked, it begins to point the way to change. Change involves uncertainty and often implies giving up what you have now for what may be and may provoke emotions of loss. Healthcare professionals, like many other professionals in organizations, often are blind to when and how these emotions appear in themselves, individually and collectively. They also often fail to take into account how these feelings are powerful feedback channels that can enhance or constrain their capacity for action.

As managed care has become more prevalent in the healthcare community, fewer seniors have been referred for inpatient rehabilitation. Instead, managed care facilities usually send enrollees to skilled nursing facilities. To respond to the changing marketplace, many acute rehabilitation providers have opened units licensed in skilled nursing in an attempt to meet this challenge. At one facility, 10 to 15% professional therapy staff left as a result of such a change. (They were not going to work in a nursing home!) Other staff members had the same emotive response and voiced their feelings but engaged in the change process. Neither of these groups was the major barrier to change for the organization. Rather, the major barrier was staff who had the same emotional response and said nothing but never truly engaged in the change effort. The latter became a major drain on the organization's effort to change.

The tools and strategies of QFD can be used to navigate these uncharted and sometimes stormy waters. Most teams and organizations that persist and remain committed to the process will be successful. Project leaders and facilitators need to be aware of these phenomena, whether they surface individually in a team member or collectively within the group.

STOP AND REFLECT

Where have you been and where are you headed? The process is summarized in Figure 7.15. You have gone to the Gemba. You captured qualitatively important data—VOCTs—using affinity diagrams and trees to send this voice; used AHP to rank the importance of that data from the customer's perspective; used questionnaires to expand this view to a larger sample of the population; and used the Kano analysis to separate

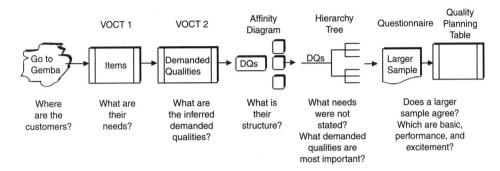

Figure 7.15. Flowchart summary of chapter 7.

the demanded qualities into basic, performance, and excitement needs. Spending time and resources to improve needs that are seen as basic does not improve customer satisfaction. Delivering what satisfies but is not expected is an opportunity to create customer excitement.

What is important? Step 1 in the QFD process (Figure 1.6) is designed to identify and reach agreement on what is important to customers. As summarized in Figure 6.20, the tools in chapter 6 identified customer segments and what customer segments are important to the organization. This chapter reviewed some practices and tools to identify what is important to those customers. Together the tools add more clarity to the organizational targets. They fleshed out details and subcomponents of the project's RNA template and ranked these details in order of importance. Next is a view of where we are headed—planning the service chain.

Chapter 8

From Customer Voice
to Design Team Voice

Upon completing this chapter, you will be able to:

- Calculate the composite importance for the customer's demanded qualities

- Calculate the priorities and performance measures for the designing requirements of the service

- Establish meaningful design targets for these measures

We are now moving to Step 2 of the QFD Process (Figure 1.6). The data captured from the survey will be placed in the Quality Planning Table. Targets for improving demanded quality and selling points will be determined, and a relative weight will be calculated for each demanded quality with respect to the total weight of the demanded qualities. The subjective demanded quality of a customer will then be translated into observable, organizational performance measures. Operational targets for these measures will be set. The tools in this chapter will translate the voice of the customer into the voice of the design team.

QUALITY PLANNING TABLE

As previously shown, the left-hand columns of the Quality Planning Table list data captured from the customers (Figure 8.1):

- Demanded qualities

- Importance ratings

- Customer competitive rankings

Demanded Qualities: the first column of the Quality Planning Table is the demanded qualities. These come from the affinity diagram and tree constructed in chapter 7. As noted earlier, the number of demanded qualities sets the level of detail for design of the service. As a rule of thumb, a maximum of 20 to 30 demanded qualities is comfortable to analyze and provides useful insight and substantial detail.

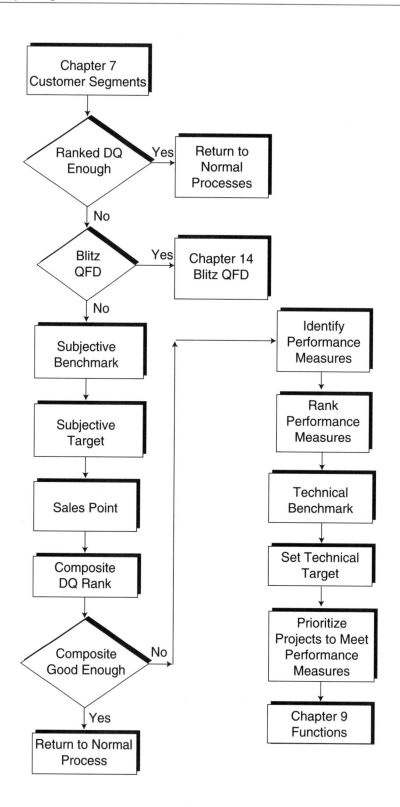

Demanded Qualities	Customer Survey Importance Rating	Our Organization	Competitor 1	Competitor 2	Competitor 3	Target	Ratio of Improvement	Sales Points	DQ Composite Importance	% Composite Importance
	B	C	C	C	C	D	E	F	G	H
1. More Comprehensive Evaluations	5	4	4	4	4	4	1	1.5	7.5	14.6
2. More Comprehensive Reports	5	4	4	4	4	5	1.25	1.5	9.38	18.2
3. Define All Findings as Pre- or Postinjury	5	4	4	4	4	5	1.25	1.5	9.38	18.2
4. Better Work Capacity Assessments	4	4	4	4	4	5	1.25	1.2	6.0	11.7
5. More MD Follow-Through with Recommendations	4	3	3	3	3	4	1.3	1.2	6.4	12.4
6. More Acceptance of Findings at Hearings	4	4	3	3	4	4	1	1.2	4.8	9.3
7. Independence From Insurers	4	4	3	4	4	4	1	1.0	4.0	7.8
8. More Understandable Reports	4	4	3	4	4	4	1	1.0	4.0	7.8
Weighted Satisfaction		136	124	136	136	154			51.5	

A

% Composite Importance

8 7 6 5 4 3

Figure 8.1. Quality Planning Table: Actual Data. The table lists demanded qualities, customer importance ratings, (Column B) and competitive comparison of delivery of these services (Columns C) captured by the surveys. Targets for improvement (Column D), ratio of improvement, (Column E) and sales point rankings (Column F) are identified. A raw composite score, a raw composite importance, (Column G) and a weighted (percent) composite importance (Column H) are calculated. The composite importance is also shown graphically.

139

Importance Ratings: the second column of the Quality Planning Table is the importance rating. In the case example, the team used actual data obtained from a customer survey to rate importance. Some organizations use data captured in the field through AHP ratings or distribution of 100 points and enter the values into the importance rating column. AHP data or distribution of 100 points data are expressed as a percentage, because the percentage is easy to see and provides ease of communication. These data also give a sense of what portion of the demanded qualities in the overall tree is captured by the table. For example, based on their AHP ranking, our eight items chosen for the Quality Planning Table represented 59 percent of the weight for the level of abstraction chosen (Figure 7.6).

Customer Competitive Rankings: the third column lists customer evaluation of the organization's service and its competitors' services. In the case example, this data was captured by a survey. Some organizations use focus groups to generate this data. As noted before, the data generated from focus groups is more qualitative in nature than is a larger survey. In addition, when an organization is unhappy with the results of a focus group, it is easier to reject the interpretation of the focus group as "a bad selection" of people than it is to reject the results from a larger sample that surveys both customers and potential customers. For this case, it was possible for the insurers to compare alternative service providers but not for the patient. If the team had initially gathered patient data, they would have to question patients who had experienced the competitors service.

The columns on the right side of the Quality Planning Table represent organizational assessments and set organizational objectives derived from the customer data. These columns include:

- Targets for improvement

- Sales points

- Composite scores

Targets for Desired Customer Satisfaction Are Selected: customer satisfaction means the customer's perceived satisfaction. A target for performance improvement for customer satisfaction is selected for each demanded quality. The target selected is influenced by:

- The organization's current performance in the eye of the customer (competitive ranking)

- The customers' opinion of the organization's service and competitions' service (competitive ranking)

- The customers' importance rating of the demanded quality (importance ratings)

- The image the organization desires to project (targets for customer satisfaction)

The targets selected consider the context of the company's strategic plan and business plan. In our example, the item *Define all findings as pre- or postinjury* had a customer importance rating of 5 and all competitors were ranked equally as 4. The team chose a target of 5 for improvement in customer satisfaction to build the perception of excellence for this demanded quality.

Ratio of Improvement: the next column is a ratio of improvement, which is calculated by dividing the target value by the current customer perception as defined by the survey.

For the item *Define all findings as pre- or postinjury,* the team set a target of 5 and current satisfaction as 4. Therefore, the ratio of improvement would be 1.25:

$$5/4 = 1.25$$

Sales Points: sales points are specific features that the organization has selected to distinguish its service from the competition. As already noted, trying to improve every aspect of service is not always practical nor even possible. Sales points are used to identify demanded qualities that have the potential to really distinguish a product or service from the competition in a particular area. Sales points in the case study were rated as 1.5, 1.2, or 1.0. The 1.5 was reserved for a demanded quality that distinguished the service from the competition; 1.2 was reserved for a demanded quality that it would be nice to have but was not critical. A value of 1.0 provided a neutral weighting. Akao (1989), one of the founders of QFD, suggests a maximum of three sales points greater than 1.0 in order to emphasize the uniqueness and increase the impact of these demanded qualities in subsequent steps of QFD and in the overall design of the service. This suggestion was overlooked by our novice QFD team.

Composite Scores: a composite or weighted score is calculated for each demanded quality. A demanded quality composite importance score is equal to the demanded quality's importance rating times the ratio of improvement times the sales point.

For the demanded quality *Define all findings as pre- or postinjury,* the customer importance rating was 5, the ratio of improvement 1.25, and the sales point 1.5, resulting in a composite score of 9.375.

$$5 \times 1.25 \times 1.5 = 9.375$$

Percent Composite Importance: For visibility and ease of communication, a percent composite importance score can be calculated for each demanded quality. This is calculated by summing the demanded quality composite score for all demanded qualities in the Quality Planning Table and then dividing each individual score by the sum total and expressing it as a percent, as shown in Figure 8.1.

$$7.5 + 9.38 + 9.38 + 6.0 + 6.4 + 4.8 + 4.0 + 4.0 = 51.46$$

The sum total of the demanded qualities composite importance score in Figure 8.1 was 51.46. The sum total 51.46 is divided into the composite score for *Define all findings as pre- or postinjury* and multiplied by 100, giving a percentage for a composite importance of 18.2 percent.

$$(9.38/51.46) \times 100 = 18.2 \text{ percent of total weight}$$

The process is repeated for all demanded qualities.

The reader might wonder why the team carried the demanded quality *Independence from insurers maintained* (Figure 8.1) into the Quality Planning Table. Although this was identified as a demanded quality during their interviews in the field, the results of the Kano model indicated that the larger customer base was somewhat indifferent to this item. Carrying the item forward may have been a function of the clinicians' core commitment to the patient/injured worker, an aversion to being seen as "working for an insurer," or another oversight by our novice team.

EXERCISE 8.1

In this exercise, data from the exercises in chapter 7 are transferred to a single location for analysis.

- If this is a learning project, select the eight most highly demanded qualities from the preceding section and enter them as the row headings in the Quality Planning Table as shown in Figure 8.1. (Use the blank form in Appendix A.) These should come from mid or lower branches of the tree but all from the same level. If this is an actual project, review the discussion about how many demanded qualities should be selected under Suggestions and Cautions, following Exercise 7.10 in chapter 7. Remember, the more demanded qualities, the more complexity and the greater number of relationships to be evaluated. The fewer the demanded qualities, the less detail in the design process.

- In the first column, list the AHP importance ratings captured in the field and the median importance rating from the customer survey.

- Enter the customer's subjective assessment of both your service and your competition.

- What does this data tell you about what is important?

- What does this data tell you about what the customers think is important?

- What does this data tell you about how your customers perceive your delivery of what is important?

- What does this data tell you about how you are perceived in delivering what is important versus your competitors?

EXERCISE 8.2

In a brief phrase, state the image/reputation your organization desires to have in the healthcare community.

- Based upon this image, what level of satisfaction should your customer have to be consistent with this desired image? It is impossible and unnecessary to have everything a 5. The target for customer satisfaction should be tempered by the importance of the demanded quality and the performance of your competition. If the item is important and every provider is currently judged as a 2, then a 3 is a significant improvement. You need only show discernible improvement in customer satisfaction. You need only be discernibly better to be ahead of the competition.

- Calculate a ratio of improvement by dividing the target by the current rating.

- Discuss how each demanded quality may work as a sales point, that is, will improving the quality distinguish you from your competitors in this area? Remember that sales points are weighted on values of 1.5, 1.2, or 1.0 and are entered into the column. Remember that Akao (1989) suggests a maximum of three sales points greater than 1.0 to emphasize the unique impact of those demanded qualities.

- Calculate an actual composite importance for each demanded quality by multiplying the customer importance score by the ratio of improvement and sales points as shown in Figure 8.1.

- Calculate the sum total for the column *Demanded Quality Composite Importance.*

- Calculate a *% Composite Importance* score for each row by dividing the demanded quality composite importance for each row by the sum of all demanded quality composite scores and multiplying by 100.

SUGGESTIONS AND CAUTIONS

Some teams and organizations find it helpful to calculate weighted satisfaction from the data about organizational competitiveness. For example, in Figure 8.1, the weighted satisfaction would be calculated by taking the customers' importance rating (5 for Row 3) and multiplying it by the customers' perception of the organization's performance (4) to yield a value of 20. This is done for each demanded quality, and then the total for the entire column is summed as shown in the figure.

$$(5 \times 4) + (5 \times 4) + (5 \times 4) + (4 \times 4) + (4 \times 3) + (4 \times 4)$$
$$+ (4 \times 4) + (4 \times 4) = 136$$

Similarly, the calculation can be carried out for competitors. The data in the case example indicated that the weighted satisfaction for the organization and Competitor 3 were the same. A weighted value can also be calculated for targets for improvement, which is a speculation by the team of the estimated customer satisfaction if all targets are met. In our example, the organization was aiming to improve from a weighted satisfaction of 136 to 154.

DEMANDED QUALITIES/PERFORMANCE MEASURES MATRIX: THE HOUSE OF QUALITY

During the first portions of the QFD process, the tools discussed have been used to assist the team and organization to identify what is important from the customers' perspective and to set targets for improvement in customer satisfaction. Although a good deal of work has been invested to clarify and identify the demanded qualities, the information is still too fuzzy to be used to design a service. In this section, we focus on defining measures of performance that will be used to predict which measures, if met, will satisfy customers. These measures will also be used to evaluate alternative ways of providing the demanded quality. The measures become predictive of the customer's level of satisfaction or dissatisfaction with the organization in providing the demanded quality.

In the QFD literature, performance measures (PM) are sometimes called quality characteristics, substitute quality characteristics, quality characteristics, requirements, or quality attributes. We will use the term *performance measure,* because the other terms may cause misdirection during this phase of the QFD process. A performance measure is a statement of what will be measured to evaluate the service's performance for a specific demanded quality. It will also be used to measure the performance of functions that will be identified later.

As noted earlier, the strength of the relationship between the demanded quality and the performance measure is the means of remapping the voice of the customer into the voice of the organization. It is here in Step 2 that the voice of the customer as a demanded quality is translated into organizational measures. Performance measures are critical to transforming how the service is delivered. In many healthcare organizations, organizational performance measures are not benchmarked for the dimensions of the service and are rarely tied back to the voice of the customer.

At least one performance measure should be identified for each demanded quality. Some teams use brainstorming exercises to generate performance measures. Another way is to use the cause-and-effect diagram (fishbone) for each demanded quality. The demanded quality is the effect, and the various performance measures then become cause (Figure 8.2). The entries in the fishbone diagram or the matrix columns answer the question "What should be measured in our system in order to predict the customer's satisfaction for demanded quality *X?*" The advantage of using the fishbone diagram is having a separate page of information for each demanded quality. Figure 8.2A is the generic fishbone, and Figure 8.2B is an example from the case study.

A glossary should also be established for each performance measure. The terms used for a performance measure are often not understood by new team members, and, as the projects move forward, the definition can change with time. A glossary must be created for the current team as well as for future users of the QFD project information. A complete glossary of terms and phrases used in the actual case are given in Appendix B. For example, the meaning of the performance measure *% Symptoms Identified* is a measure of a ratio for all the symptoms identified and discussed in the evaluation process to every symptom that has been previously recorded. Every statement expressing a change in capability, feeling, confidence, and so on made by the patient is considered a symptom. The percentage of symptoms identified and listed in the report as industrial or nonindustrial to total symptoms recorded over the course of injury or reported as not being identified by us, by treating physicians, or by case managers at one month follow-up will be used as the performance measure *% Symptoms Identified.* The experience of the team has been that if symptoms were not categorized in the report, the insurance case managers would call and ask about them.

The number of demanded qualities entered into the rows sets the level of detail. The complexity of analysis is the product of the number of rows and columns, a context for complexity, that is, the number of relationships that need to be evaluated. The number of performance measures entered in the columns will also determine the complexity of the matrix. The number of columns should be kept in the range of less than 30. Usually, the number of performance measures exceeds the number of demanded qualities.

Our experience in healthcare is that most measures in healthcare delivery have evolved out of habit or previous needs, not by design (Institute of Medicine 1985). In

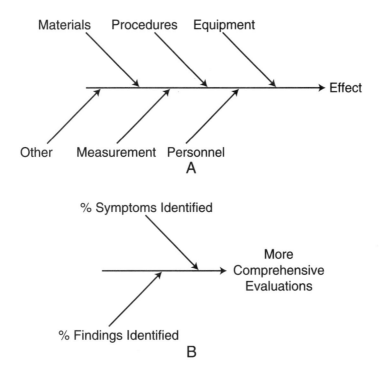

Figure 8.2. Fishbone cause-and-effect diagram. (A) Fishbone cause and effect is a very basic tool to identify contributing factors and contributing causes.
(B) The demanded quality is the effect, and the various performance measures then become cause. The entries in the fishbone diagram or the matrix columns answer the question "What should be measured in our system in order to predict the customer's satisfaction for demanded quality *X*?"

most processes, key functions and critical tasks are not clearly identified except in critical care areas, such as code blue, ICU, and so on. Immediate feedback as to how the service is being delivered is often lacking. Therefore, a small number of performance measures, if well chosen, can result in substantial improvement in the level of most services. In our example, Figure 8.3, 10 performance measures were entered into the matrix.

If the list of potential performance measures generated by the team becomes very large, the affinity diagram can be used to raise the level of abstraction and thus reduce the number under consideration. In general, the same level of abstraction should be included in all competitive ranking and evaluative matrices. Performance measures that are selected are entered into the columns of the Demanded Qualities/Performance Measures Matrix (Figure 8.3).

Rows—Demanded Qualities: the demanded qualities from Step 1 in the Quality Planning Table are entered into rows of the matrix along with their relative importance ratings.

Columns—Performance Measures: performance measures are entered into the columns of the matrix. There should be at least one performance measure for each demanded quality. Try to avoid pass/fail measures, because these make it more difficult to select quality.

Demanded Qualities/ Performance Measures Matrix	DQs % Composite Importance	% Symptoms Identified	% Findings Identified	% Treatments Identified	% Findings Linked to Observable Data	% Findings Separated into Industrial or Nonindustrial	% Job Requirements Simulated and Tested	% Capacities and Impairments Quantified	% of Workers' Treating MDs Included in Process	% Returned to Work	Number Unexplained Inconsistencies
Direction of Improvement		↑	↑	↑	↑	↑	↑	↑	↑	↑	↓
1. More Comprehensive evaluations	14.60	●	●	◐	○						
3. Definition of All Findings as Pre- or Postinjury	18.20	●			●	●					
4. Better Work Capacity Assessments	11.70		○	◐			●	●			●
5. More MD Follow-Through with Recommendations	12.40				◐	◐	●		●	●	◐
6. More Acceptance of Findings at Hearings	9.30	●	◐		●	●	◐	◐			●
7. Independence from Insurers Maintained	7.80	◐		●	●		◐	◐	◐	◐	
8. More Understandable Reports	7.80				●			◐			◐
Absolute Importance		402.3	171.0	149.1	369.5	354.9	268.2	180.0	135.0	135.0	249.6
Relative Importance		16.7%	7.1%	6.2%	15.3%	14.7%	11.1%	7.5%	5.6%	5.6%	10.3%
Selected		Y	N	N	Y	Y	Y	N	Y	N	Y
Target		100			100	100	100		100		0

● Strong Relationship   ◐ Medium Relationship   ○ Weak Relationship

Figure 8.3. Demanded Qualities/Performance Measures Matrix. This matrix is often referred to as the *House of Quality.* It compares the relationship between demanded qualities and performance measures (measurable quality characteristics) for these. Cell by cell, the strength of each performance measure's (columns) ability to predict each demanded quality (rows) is rated as ● strong, ◐ medium, ○ weak, or blank. The strength of the relationships within the cell is then weighted by multiplying it by the importance rating of the demanded quality. Those columns that are strongly correlated with demanded qualities are selected to be carried to the next matrix. Specific units of measure for each performance measure and targets are identified for these measures.

Source: Figure and calculations done with software from QualiSoft, 4652 Patrick Rd., West Bloomfield, Mich. 48233, qualisoft@aol.com. Demo available www.qualisoft.com.

In the case study, *% Symptoms Identified* was one performance measure for the demanded quality *More Comprehensive Evaluations* (Figure 8.2B).

Strength of Each Relationship: the strength of each cell in the matrix is identified for the column's ability to predict satisfaction for the demanded quality in the row. This is done by asking the question, "If you know the value for the performance measure X, how well will it predict customer satisfaction for demanded quality Y?" The team uses four options to rank the strength of the relationship:

●	A strong relationship with a value of	9
◕	A medium relationship with a value of	3
○	A weak relationship with a value of	1
	No relationship with a value of	0

The filled circle, quarter-filled circle, and empty circle, provide for easy visibility and communication. The patterns that develop will be used to check the structure of the matrix. It is very helpful to put a small dot in the cells for which the team has identified no relationship so that the team knows the cell has been evaluated.

The use of the 9, 3, 1 scale can force the properties of the Pareto principle, that is, that most of the customers' perception of value comes from a few items. The assumption is that if you deliver the most critical demanded qualities (e.g., 20 percent), you will satisfy most of the customers' desire (e.g., 80 percent).

In completing the matrix, keep in mind that not everything is related. If you are not sure a relationship exists, do not assume a weak relationship. Instead, put a question mark there and, after further discussion, replace it with the appropriate symbol.

The goal in the matrix is to have at least one moderate or higher performance measure for each demanded quality. A row with no strong or moderate relationship with a performance measure, such as blank or all dots, means that demanded quality is being ignored in the service because there is no strong predictor being measured in service performance for that demanded quality. Alternatively, a blank column, such as a column that does not strongly or moderately correspond to a row, indicates that the organization may be wasting resources by designing a function to produce and measure an outcome that does not address a customer or regulatory need.

Our experience is that the overcollection of data is a very common phenomenon in healthcare. We see many healthcare organizations that collect data that are not strongly or moderately related to customers' satisfaction or regulatory requirements. We also note that, even when data are collected for measures that do correlate with customer satisfaction, the data are not fed back in a timely manner to the people who actually deliver the service in a way to reinforce desirable or inhibit undesirable performance behavior. Much of the data collected is by retrospective chart review after the patient has been sent home. This is like checking a packing list for completeness after the order has been shipped and received.

In the study, both *% Symptoms Identified* and *% Findings Identified* were rated as being strongly predictive of satisfying the demanded quality *More Comprehensive Evaluations.* The column *% Returned to Work* as a performance measure was not felt to have a particular relationship to this demanded quality.

Weighting Each Cell: each cell is weighted by multiplying its ranking (9, 3, 1, or 0) by the relative importance rating for the row. For the demanded quality *More Comprehensive Evaluations,* the percent composite rating of 14.5 would be multiplied by 9, equaling 131.4 for that cell.

$$14.5 \times 9 = 131.4$$

Each cell in the matrix is similarly weighted.

Weighing Columns: The sum of each column is calculated (Absolute importance). The sum of all the columns combined is calculated and the weight of each column is divided by the total column weight and multiplied by 100 (Relative importance expressed as %). Highly weighted performance measures are selected.

The five highest weighted characteristics and the measure *"% of Workers' Treating MDs included in Process"* were selected as the performance measure to be carried to the next step. Although the weight of *"% of Workers' Treating MDs included in Process"* was only slightly more than half that for the next highest ranking attribute chosen (5.6% versus 10.3%), the measure was chosen from Kano questionnaire data. The data indicated that the demanded quality *"More MDs Follow-Through with Recommendations"* had the potential to produce customer excitement and *"% of Workers' Treating MDs included in Process"* was seen as a potential measurable dimension of that quality and was carried forward.

Selecting Targets for Performance Measures: During this step, the team begins to plan the actual service. The team sets targets for design requirements and prioritizes these for the service. When benchmarking data are available from competing services, these data can be incorporated at this level. Performance measures must include units of measure. Try to avoid pass/fail measures. These make it more difficult to select the best direction for improvement later in the design process.

This matrix has identified critical performance measures and associated targets. The output of this analysis (the House of Quality Analysis) is the selection of a few critical, new, and important performance measures. This matrix then can serve as a living document for the remainder of the QFD process and also for CQI and future design projects.

The careful reader will note that in the case study, the demanded quality *More Comprehensive Reports,* which appears in the Quality Planning Table, does not appear in the Demanded Qualities/Performance Measures Matrix in Figure 8.3. When the team ranked performance measures with respect to this demanded quality, almost all the cells had a very strong relationship. This pattern persisted even after multiple discussions. Rows that correlate very strongly with *all* performance measures may actually be a reliability or safety item or may include other demanded qualities from a lower level of affinity grouping. Including such items in this matrix can skew the subsequent matrix calculations, so the team dropped the item.

CHECKING THE QUALITY DEPLOYMENT MATRIX
FOR WEAKNESS AND OVERSIGHT

There are ten checks (Nakui 1991) that should be performed to assure the most useful matrix for analysis. The symbols used facilitate seeing patterns, just like the yearly *Consumer Reports* for automobiles. It is easy to pick the best car just by scanning the patterns presented. The method introduced for identifying the performance measures minimizes the likelihood of failing some of these tests (Figure 8.4).

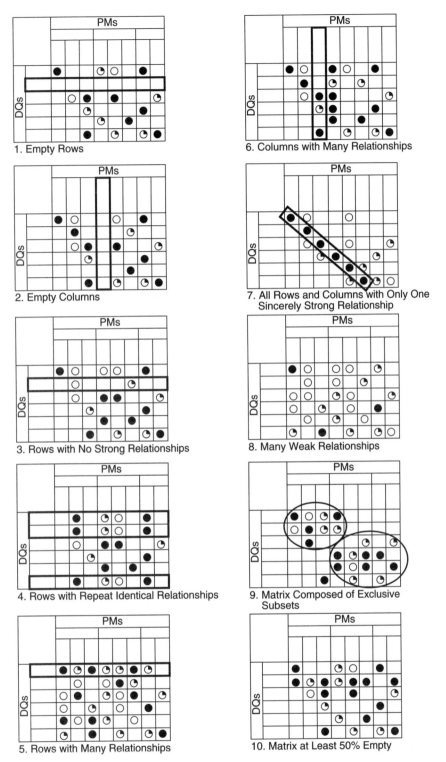

Figure 8.4. Checking the Quality Deployment Matrix for weaknesses and oversights. There are ten checks that should be performed to assure the most useful matrix for analysis. A detailed description of each is included in the text.

1. Empty Rows: if a demanded quality has no performance measure entries in its row, then there will be no data to predict the customer satisfaction for this demanded quality. If the demanded quality is not very important, this may not be an issue. Removing this demanded quality is one way to reduce the size of the matrix.

2. Empty Columns: if a performance measure does not relate to any demanded quality, why collect the measure? It is a waste of time and resources. If this performance measure is included only because it has always been used in the past, then it should now be removed. If the performance measure is critical for satisfying a federal requirement, then the measure must be performed but the matrix will give it zero importance. A special set of columns should be set to the right of the matrix as Must Do. They will be in this matrix and possibly others but will not be used in the analysis.

3. Rows with No Strong Relationships: if this is even a modestly important demanded quality, the customer may be unhappy because there is no effective way to predict customer satisfaction. At least one strong performance measure should be found. If the demanded quality is not very important, this is not a problem.

4. Rows with Repeat Identical Relationships: if multiple rows have the same patterns of relationships, these rows may be the same demanded quality with different words. This will create a double or triple accounting for the importance of the related performance measures. If the rows are the same, remove the redundant rows. If they are different, then leave them in the matrix.

5. Rows with Many Relationships: if a row has many strong and medium relationships, then that row may be at a higher level of abstraction than the other rows. Go back to the affinity diagram and check to see if this demanded quality is actually a group heading. The same pattern will exist if cost, reliability, or safety has been made a demanded quality. These should be removed from this matrix and used later or in other analyses.

6. Columns with Many Relationships: if a column has too many relationships, it may be at a higher level of abstraction than the other columns. Go back to the affinity diagram and check to see if this performance measure is actually a group heading. The same pattern will exist if cost, reliability, or safety has been made a performance measure. These should be removed from this matrix and used later or in other analyses.

7. All Rows and Columns with Only One Strong Relationship: if in the whole matrix there are very few entries other than the one strong relationship in each row and column, the matrix is not going to provide very many insights. This means that the demanded qualities and the performance measures are really the same thing. This is more likely to happen when the team—rather than the customer—generates the demanded qualities.

8. Many Weak Relationships: if the team is very conservative, they will see some predictive value for every performance measure. The matrices in QFD can be viewed as a variation on the Pareto chart. One of the purposes of the Pareto chart is to identify the critical few. Including many weak relationships dilutes the sensitivity of the analysis.

9. Matrix Composed of Exclusive Subsets: if the rows and columns can be rearranged into separate and distinct blocks, these blocks can be considered as smaller, separate matrices. This will make the analysis much easier.

10. Matrix at Least 50% Empty: again, from the perspective of Pareto, not everything is important. This is usually the outcome when the team is being overly cautious and seeing more relationships than are necessary.

EXERCISE 8.3

- Enter demanded qualities from the Quality Planning Table in the rows of the Demanded Qualities/Performance Measures Matrix (blank sample in Appendix A).

- Enter Composite Importance Ratings from the Quality Planning Table in the first column.

- Generate a list of performance measures for these demanded qualities. If the list is too long, use affinity groupings to raise the level of abstraction.

- Enter the performance measures in the columns of the table.

- For each column and row ask, "If you knew the value for performance measure *X,* how well would it predict the customer's level of satisfaction for demanded quality *Y?*

- Determine the strength of the predictive relationship between each performance measure and demanded quality as

  ●   Strong predictive relationship

  ◖   Medium predictive relationship

  ○   Weak predictive relationship

  •   No predictive relationship

- Each important demanded quality must have at least one performance measure with at least a medium relationship. A strong relationship is preferred.

- Before calculations, check for patterns in the matrix. Look for signs of an unbalanced matrix.

- Each cell is weighted by multiplying its relationship—● strong, ◖ medium, ○ weak, (blank or •) none—by the demanded composite importance rating. The weighted importance for each performance measure is determined by summing the columns, and the total weight of all the columns is calculated. The percentage importance for each column is then expressed as a percentage of the total.

USING BENCHMARKING DATA TO CHECK INTERNAL CONSISTENCY

Performance measures can be displayed with the subjective data from the Quality Planning Table on the right, as shown in Figure 8.5. When benchmarking data are available,

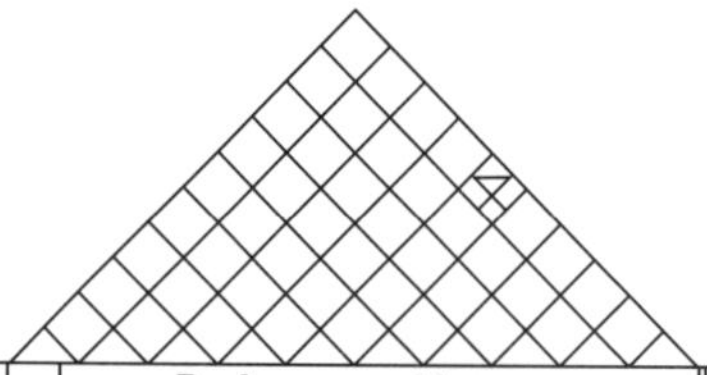

House of Quality	Customer Importance	% Symptoms Identified	% Findings Identified	% Treatments Identified	% Findings Linked to Observable Data	% Findings Separated into Industrial or Nonindustrial	% Job Requirements Simulated and Tested	% Capacities and Impairments Quantified	% of Workers' Treating MDs Included in Process	% Returned to Work	Number Unexplained Inconsistencies	Our Organization	Competitor 1	Competitor 2	Competitor 3	Target	Ratio of Improvement	Sales Points	DQ Composite Importance	% DQ Composite Importance
Direction of Improvement		↑	↑	↑	↑	↑	↑	↑	↑	↑	↓									
Demanded Qualities 1. More Comprehensive Evaluations	5	●	●	◔	○	✓	✓	✓	✓	✓	✓	4	4	4	4	4	1.0	1.5	7.5	**14.6**
3. Definition of All Findings as Pre- or Postinjury	5	●	✓	✓	●	●	✓	✓	✓	✓	✓	4	4	4	4	5	1.3	1.5	9.4	**18.2**
4. Better Work Capacity Assessments	5	✓	○	◔	✓	✓	●	●	✓	✓	●	4	4	4	4	5	1.3	1.2	6.0	**11.7**
5. More MD Follow-Through with Recommendations	4	✓	✓	✓	◔	◔	●	✓	●	●	◔	3	3	3	3	4	1.3	1.2	6.4	**12.4**
6. More Acceptance of Findings at Hearings	4	●	◔	✓	●	●	◔	◔	✓	✓	●	4	3	3	4	4	1.0	1.2	4.8	**9.3**
7. Independence from Insurers Maintained	4	◔	✓	●	●	✓	◔	◔	◔	◔	✓	4	3	4	4	4	1.0	1.0	4.0	**7.8**
8. More Understandable Reports	4	✓	✓	✓	✓	●	✓	◔	✓	✓	◔	4	3	4	4	4	1.0	1.0	4.0	**7.8**
Benchmarking Data																				
Organizational Difficulty																				
Absolute Importance		402.3	171.0	149.1	369.5	354.9	268.2	180.0	135.0	135.0	249.6									
Relative Importance		16.7%	7.1%	6.2%	15.3%	14.7%	11.1%	7.5%	5.6%	5.6%	10.3%									
Selected		Y	N	N	Y	Y	Y	N	Y	N	Y									
Target		100			100	100	100		100		0									

● Strong Relationship
◔ Medium Relationship
○ Weak Relationship

⊙ Strong Positive
○ Positive
Negative
× Strong Negative

Figure 8.5. Roof of the House of Quality. Traditionally, a roof was added to identify synergies and contradictions hence the name House of Quality. ✓ means no relationship.

they are placed at the base of the columns for the performance measures. With measurable benchmarking data, we are not only able to rank performance measure, but we can also compare our current service with the competitions' service. In contrast to the survey data, benchmarking is usually called objective benchmarking because defined metrics applied by neutral parties are used to do the measuring. The results help set your standard for performance.

The results of objective benchmarking can also be used to check and validate the strong predictive relationships in the matrix. Any cell that has a strong predictive relationship should be the intersection of a row with high subjective and competitive rankings and a column with constant objective benchmarking data. The customer's subjective ordering of the performance of the market services should match the organization's objective ordering of the competing services. If they do not, the strong relationship placed in the cell was not warranted or the performance measure is not measuring the correct aspect of the service. In the case study, benchmarking data was not available so this activity was not carried out. To illustrate how this activity is used in the process, we present another example (Figure 8.6). In this hypothetical case, the demanded qualities, performance measures, and benchmarking data are as follows.

The Demanded Qualities

Fast evaluation: Referral sources want assessments done as soon as possible.

Helpful: Customers want their questions answered quickly.

Short time in the system: Time from entry in the system to exit is short.

Easy to control: Healthcare administrator wants an easy way to manage the system.

The Performance Measures

Time, time from the beginning of the actual evaluation of the patient until the evaluation is complete: The arrow down means fewer days are more desirable.

Hours, total number of hours per day the help line is available to answer questions: The arrow up means more hours are more desirable.

Staffing, total number of staff available for assessment: The bull's-eye means a specific value is best because more staff could reduce the time to complete assessments, but a smaller staff is easier to manage.

Subjective Data

Data is captured from customer questionnaires.

Benchmarking

Us is our organization.

Them 1 is the AZY Corp.

Them 2 is the Heavenly Care Village.

Only strong relationships indicated by the ● are included in this example. We will show how these relationships compare to rank the subjective data (surveys) and the objective data (benchmarks).

Looking at the shaded row and column, we see that the row and column are in agreement. *Fast Evaluation* benchmarking data shows that the *Time* from the beginning of the assessment to completion is 4 days for our organization, 5 days for Them 1, and 15 days for Them 2. The subjective data shows 5, 4, and 1 for *Fast Evaluation* for Us, Them 1, and Them 2, respectively. The survey results are consistent with the benchmarking data (a 5 is very good, and a 1 is poor).

The performance measure *Time* is not doing as well for the third demanded quality *Short Time in System.* The benchmarking data for *Time* indicate that the measure is not a good one for the demanded quality *Short Time in System*. The strong relationship initially entered into the matrix (the measure in the column that strongly predicted satisfaction for the row) is not consistent with benchmarking data and the subjective ranking.

There are small differences in subjective ranking, but big differences in the benchmarking data. The subjective ratings from the customers are 4, 4, and 5; while the times are 4, 5, and 15 days. The customer is saying that Them 2 is best while the technical benchmarking is saying we are the best. *Time* is a poor performance measure for the demanded quality *Short Time in System*, which can be explained by the fact that time for evaluation is only a small part of the total time in the system.

The performance measure *Hours* is not a good predictor for the demanded quality *Helpful*. The organization that offers a help line all day long is not considered the best. There could be some other measures, such as courteousness, that are shadowing the effect of the hours available. Possibly, *Hours* should not be used. This suggests that there is another demanded quality leading to at least one other performance measure.

There are two reasons why a performance measure should have a target value rather than a smaller- or larger-is-best measure. Sometimes one row has a demanded quality requiring a larger value for the performance measure, and another row has a demanded quality requiring a smaller value for the performance measure. In this situation, a specific value is best. This may be a good time to use the Theory of Inventive Problem Solving (TRIZ, see Appendix D) to remove the contradiction.

If no competing services currently exist, there is no means to evaluate alternatives. The most highly weighted performance measure is not necessarily the one to improve. If the competitor's performance measure benchmark scores are much poorer than yours, you should consider improving the next highest ranked performance measure, since improving the one you already excel in may not provide the greatest opportunity for improvement from the customers' perspective. Do not blindly allocate resources to the performance measure with the largest number, because it may not be the most important for capturing a larger share of the market.

SYNERGY AND CONFLICTS

Care must also be taken in selecting target values, because the performance of one performance measure may impact another in the current system. There are times when improving one performance measure in a service may conflict with and actually degrade another performance measure. These interrelationships need to be considered when designing the service. For example, both performance measures *% Symptoms Identified* and *% Findings Separated into Industrial or Nonindustrial* have targets of 100 percent. These assessments would be performed by multiple observers. *Number Unexplained Inconsistencies* has a target of 0 (Figure 8.3). Increasing the level of detail for the former two performance measures increases potential conflicts with reaching the latter performance measure. With more detail in the former measures, there is more opportunity for inconsistencies. This would have a negative effect on reaching the target of 0 unexplained inconsistencies between observers. Conflicts like this need to be considered, and attempts to design measures to decrease or eliminate conflicts should be explored.

Traditionally, conflicts were illustrated by putting a roof on the Demanded Qualities/Performance Measures Matrix, hence the name House of Quality (Figure 8.5). Each cell of the roof is the intersection of two performance measures. Relationships between performance measures can be found by asking the question, "If performance measure *X* is improved, will it help or hinder performance measure *Z?*" Negative relationships represent constraints. Five symbols for the interactions are used:

⊙   Strong positive

●   Positive

✗✗   Negative

✗   Strong negative

We can also check for synergies and conflicts by using a matrix of performance measures versus performance measures (Figure 8.7). This matrix should be used only when small changes are to be made to the existing system. To illustrate this, we will use the benchmarking examples from Figure 8.6; but an additional performance measure has been added, *Total Time in the System (TTS)*.

Begin completing the table in Figure 8.7 from the rows in Figure 8.6. The cells in each row are evaluated by asking the question, "If I improve the row, will it enhance or hinder improvement of the column?" Enhancing is indicated by one or two plus symbols, and hindering is indicated by one or two minus symbols. A blank cell means there was no effect upon the corresponding row and column.

If the *Time* to complete the assessment is reduced, it will reduce the total time in the system. But reducing the *Total Time in the System* may not have an effect on the *Time* to complete the assessment if the majority of time in the system is scheduling the evaluation and generating a comprehensive report. Often the synergy is bidirectional but not always. This matrix is particularly useful because it will detect nonsymmetric synergies. A nonsymmetric synergy is one in which improving *X* has an effect on *Y*, which is different than improving *Y* having an effect on *X*. This is not a frequent occurrence, but it does occur. Performance measures have an effect on each other.

EXERCISE 8.4

Compare the percentages for weighted importance of the performance measures in your matrix. For those that rank high, define units of measures and set targets. Check for internal consistency in rows and columns.

EXERCISE 8.5

Check for positive and negative synergy in your example.

EXERCISE 8.6

Validate the strength of relationships. In any cell where there is a strong relationship between the performance measure and the demanded quality, there should be agreement with customer evaluation and any available benchmarking. Compare the percentages for weighted importance for the performance measures in your matrix. Check for internal consistency in rows and columns. For those that rank high, define units of measures and set targets.

		PM			Subjective Benchmark		
		Time	Hours	Staffing	Us	Them 1	Them 2
		↓	↑	◉			
DQ	Fast Evaluation	●		●	5	4	2
	Helpful		●		2	4	1
	Short Time in System	●			4	4	5
	Easy to Control			●			
Objective Benchmark	Us	4 days	24 hours	6			
	Them 1	5 days	8 hours	8			
	Them 2	15 days	10 hours	2			

Figure 8.6. Matrix for internal consistency with benchmarking data when benchmarking data is available. It can be checked for consistency with strongly rated measures in the matrix by comparing objective data, the rating of the measure for the demanded quality, and the customer's objective perceptions of whether the quality is being satisfied or not.

EXERCISE 8.7

Select target values. An organization's target values are a function of the current capacity of the organization and the competitiveness of its environment. The following should be considered:

- How important is the performance measure?
- If benchmarking data is available, how does the organization compare to the competition on this measure?
- How does the performance measure relate to the corporate image?
- What are the organization's technical capabilities for delivering the measure?
- What resources are available?
- In what direction do you think the competition is moving with respect to this measure?

The team can now select which aspect of service improvement will be furnished with money and/or staff. A row called *Implementation* will have a *Yes* if the team has chosen to rank a project delivering this measure or a *No* if the team decides the measure will not be worked on at this time. A *?* can always be used to indicate that further discussion is needed.

++ Very Positive Synergy			PM			
+ Positive Synergy – Negative Synergy – – Very Negative Synergy No Relationship			TTS	Time	Hours	Staffing
			↓	↓	↑	◎
PM	TTS	↓				
	Time	↓	+			
	Hours	↑				
	Staffing	◎				

Figure 8.7. Synergy Matrix. A Synergy Matrix is more useful for identifying synergies and contradictions than traditional "roof". Synergies are rated as positive, very positive, no relationship, negative, or very negative.

MULTIPLE CUSTOMERS

In healthcare, there are two different structures for multiple customers.

Simultaneous Multiple Customers: different customer segments must be satisfied by the same system/service. The needs of the different groups may or may not be in conflict, but they will all feel the impact of one system used to provide the services. For example, hospital care of the elderly must satisfy the needs of the patient, family, Medicare, and so on. It is useful in understanding the conflicts and similarities to use the Synergy Matrix for every pair of customer segments. The definition of the cell's content changes a little. Cells are evaluated by asking the question, "If we satisfy the demanded quality in the row for Customer Segment A, will it enhance or hinder our effort to satisfy the demanded quality in the column for Customer Segment B?" Having no effect is also a response.

Exclusive Multiple Customers: these customers must be satisfied by completely different systems/services. The system for hospice patients need not be the same as the system for emergency patients. It may be possible to design one system for both, but it is not necessary.

For hospitals, there are multiple customers: the patient or end consumer, the insurer, the payer of the insurance (which may or may not be the patient, and may include the government and employers), and other healthcare professionals such as physicians. The team in the chapter 4 example did not have the opportunity to interview groups of patients. However, over a period of time, as patients were evaluated, injured workers were interviewed, data pooled, and a Demanded Qualities/Performance Measures Matrix constructed (Figure 8.8).

First a group of injured workers/customers were asked why they wanted the service. After interviewing a series of those workers, the team noted a number of responses that were consistently present. The next 15 injured workers being evaluated were asked to rank the importance of each of their demanded qualities using AHP pairwise comparisons. Their individual responses were averaged by using a geometric mean to obtain importance ratings for their demanded qualities. This generated demanded qualities and importance data, from which the team developed the matrix in Figure 8.8. Ideally, each customer segment is interviewed in the field by *going to the Gemba* and identifying demanded qualities for each customer group.

Injured Workers' Demanded Qualities/Performance Measures Matrix	AHP Importance Score	% Symptoms Identified	% Findings Identified	% Treatments Identified	% Findings Linked to Observable Data	% Findings Separated into Industrial or Nonindustrial	% Job Requirements Simulated and Tested	% Capacities and Impairments Quantified	% of Workers' Treating MDs Included in Process	% Returned to Work	Number Unexplained Inconsistencies
		Performance Measures									
Direction of Improvement		↑	↑	↑	↑	↑	↑	↑	↑	↑	↓
Demanded Qualities 1. I want something to make me more normal.	8.60	◔	◔	●			○			○	
2. Show me how to live with my limitations.	14.00	◔		◔			○	●		○	
3. I want relief from pain.	40.00	◔	◔	●					●		
4. I want to be able to return to recreational activities.	3.00	◔						●			
5. I want understandable answers.	8.90	◔	●	◔	●	●		◔	◔		
6. I want to be listened to.	15.00	●		●	◔						●
7. I want to be treated like a human being.	5.00	●		◔	◔						●
8. I want to get back to work.	4.90			●			●	◔	◔		◔
9. I want compensation for my injuries.	1.50	●						●			
Absolute Importance		417.0	225.9	700.2	140.1	80.10	66.70	207.9	401.4	22.60	194.7
Relative Importance		17.0%	9.2%	28.5%	5.7%	3.3%	2.7%	8.5%	16.3%	0.9%	7.9%

● Strong Relationship ◔ Medium Relationship ○ Weak Relationship

Figure 8.8. Injured Workers' Matrix. The Demanded Qualities/Performance Measures Matrix for injured workers.

Compare the performance measures for the workers in Figure 8.3 and those for injured workers in Figure 8.8. By including the workers' demanded qualities in the matrix, two performance measures emerged that were not identified directly by the insurer customer segment as particularly important, *% Treatments Identified* and *% Workers' Treating MDs Included in Process.* The latter had already been identified as a performance measure for the demanded quality *More MD Follow-Through with*

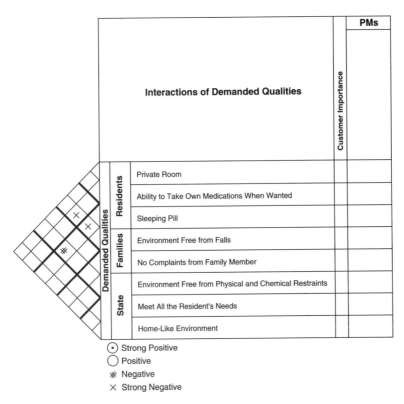

Figure 8.9. Side roof: Multiple Customer Matrix. Synergies and contradictions as a way of identifying customer segments.

Recommendations, which had been identified in the Kano questionnaire as having the potential to create excitement. This is an example of robustness of QFD when the tools are used appropriately to uncover important measures of performance for qualities demanded by customers.

A *side roof,* or demanded qualities versus demanded qualities synergy table, sometimes uncovers conflicts between different customer segments. If the team had demanded qualities for the patient, their family, and the state agencies, they could look at the synergy between the requirements (Figure 8.9):

- A *resident* wants to be able to take his or her own medications when he or she wants. A resident wants to be able to have something to take to sleep if they are having trouble sleeping.

- *Families* want an environment free from falls; however, taking sleeping pills increases the chance of falling, hence the strong negative correlation between the demanded qualities *Ability to Take Own Medications When Wanted* and *Sleeping Pill* and the demanded quality *Environment Free from Falls.*

- *Federal/state regulations* classify sleeping pills in the same category as a chemical restraint, hence the negative interaction between the demanded quality *Sleeping Pill* and the demanded quality *Environment Free from Physical and Chemical Restraints.*

In this example, the different customer segments were known. When strong conflicts are noted between demanded qualities thought to be from one customer segment, then it is possible that there are really demanded qualities from the different customer segments included in the matrix. This should be evaluated by revisiting the customer characteristics.

SUGGESTIONS AND CAUTIONS

As we have noted, in some organizations the team will stop after a particular step in the QFD process and will return to their existing process to implement change based on what they have learned to that point. Some organizations find that all they need to do with QFD tools is identify a few critical performance measures and then return to their traditional process. This, however, should be done as a positive step, a conscious decision designed to improve the service. In Figure 2.9, our archetypal model for change, this would be represented as moving from Point 2 to Point 3. It should not be done to adopt the path of least resistance, which is represented as moving from Point 2 back to Point 1.

When teams are working on the Demanded Qualities/Performance Measures Matrix, there is a tendency to gloss over the performance measures and jump to solutions without considering the importance of the performance measures in identifying and monitoring the key functions for delivering those measures, potential failure modes, and critical tasks. This can be a serious mistake. Functions, Failure Modes, and Critical Tasks are addressed in later chapters.

In healthcare, setting targets for performance measures can be a challenge. We have noticed a tendency for healthcare professionals, particularly physicians, to provide lots of anecdotal information as to why such and such a target is not possible. When key assumptions and expectations that underlie their experience are challenged by the rankings and they are asked to make commitments to these targets, or even the process itself, responded of denial and anger are easily provoked. A common and usually unconscious behavior is to make problems increasingly complicated by saying "yes, but . . . ." The net result is that the task begins to appear so overwhelming that no new action is possible. The reinforcing payoff for the "yes, but . . ." behavior is the avoidance of the risk that accompanies change (see Appendix G for more comments on resistance and performance measures). Goldratt (1990) has commented on layers of resistance or inertia that constrain change and the types of conversations that manifest at each stage:

1. That is not our problem (blindness or denial).

2. This is not the right direction to look for a solution (denial).

3. That is the solution (what I want is . . .).

4. There would be negative effects if we did it (yes, but).

5. There are these obstacles to . . . (yes, but).

6. I am afraid to . . . (underlying emotion).

If there is not some "stretch" in setting targets, the probability of substantially improving service is decreased. If you always reach for the nearest object, you will never reach one that is farther away. On the other hand, if you set out to reach the object that is a stretch, you have the opportunity to reduce or modify your reach to a nearer object if necessary. Remember, after deployment, it is more costly to add the infrastructure required to reach the targets beyond those of the initial design.

In general, our experience is that healthcare providers collect far too much data that have weak relationships to customer or regulatory satisfaction. The excess data then becomes noise that obscures critical relationships that do exist. Too much data and too many targets present unclear targets and confusing feedback, which are fertilizer for moods of resignation and resentment. Rather than enhancing the clarity of the target and the usefulness of feedback, too much measuring not strongly linked to the target obscures the target and degrades performance rather than enhancing it. In some cases, the collection of data has itself become the target, without any link to the environment. Often much of the data collected were added at some point in the organization's history to address a particular problem and were not discarded when the problem was resolved, or an additional measure was added because the problem failed to be resolved. The *as is* system often evolves as a collage rather than by design. It resembles the Winchester House in San Jose, CA, with stairways that go nowhere and doors that do not open. The rooms were designed for the appearance of the room and not the function of the whole house.

When weighting the strength of each relationship in the matrix, it is helpful to record both controversial and critical discussions and add them to a journal of important notes. It is useful if the entries are cross-referenced.

STOP AND REFLECT

This section adds even more clarity to the target and sets the code for the service's RNA. First, a finite set of demanded qualities is identified and selected based on data captured from the customer environment. This allows the team to focus its actions and thus increases the chance of success. These targets are feed-forward loops (Figure 3.4).

Next, performance measures are identified. These provide a compass by which to navigate. These measures provide feedback loops.

What is important? This step in the QFD process identifies and generates agreement on what must be measured to ensure delivery of what is identified as important to customers. To this point, we have assessed an organization's readiness (capacities stored in an organization's DNA) and we have identified detailed targets for the delivery of future services (the service RNA). We have identified performance measures that will be used to identify and adjust actions. We are now ready to identify key and necessary actions to reach the targets.

Chapter 9

Key Functions

Upon completing this chapter, you will be able to:

- Identify key functions that influence Performance Measures or Demanded Qualities

FUNCTION DEPLOYMENT

A function describes the overall purpose of a process or subprocess. As used here, a function is a set of actions or series of actions that must occur to satisfy a demanded quality or influence a performance measure without necessarily identifying the detailed steps and rules that are required. The latter are considered tasks and are identified later in Task Deployment.

For example, *Schedule entire evaluation prior to workers' arrival* was identified as a key function in the case study (Figure 9.1). This function would include multiple tasks, such as reviewing medical records, reviewing a completed survey of items filled out by the injured worker, and so on, in order to identify problems, specialists needed, special tests, and so on.

The function of the service is to satisfy the demanded qualities by achieving the performance measure's target value. In the service industry, unlike in manufacturing, the result of a function is not necessarily an artifact or a thing. The result frequently cannot be stored and is more difficult to measure and account for. One of the goals of Function Deployment is to make the key functions of the service process more visible and, therefore, easier to evaluate, measure, and design.

In biological systems, there is often a key step in each process that influences overall rate and throughput of the process. In biochemistry, this is called the rate-limiting step. One of the goals of functional analysis is to identify such steps in the service line, as introducing change at this step can enhance or constrain the overall process. Such steps are also points to incorporate reinforcing and balancing feedback from results of the process. The incorporation of reinforcing and inhibiting feedback around important performance measures for the service is key to designing a self-organizing and self-regulating delivery system and reducing variation. Incorporating reinforcing and balancing feedback is a key strategy for overcoming the challenge of differentiation and integration—the conflict of the parts versus the whole every system faces. Feedback

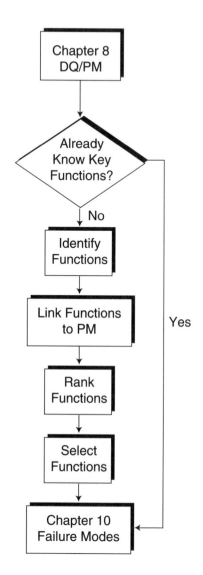

linked to the overall target of the function or the process helps overcome our biological tendency to focus on the task before us (short-term) versus the final destination (long-term). This is discussed further under New Process Deployment (Step 5).

PERFORMANCE MEASURES/FUNCTIONS MATRIX
OR DEMANDED QUALITIES/FUNCTIONS MATRIX

To define functions, the team can use the brainstorming process to list functions currently in the service or anticipated to be in the service. A single-level fishbone tool can also be used with a demanded quality or performance measure at the head and functions as the input to the bones.

A function is a required performance action described by an active verb and a noun (measurable) without identifying the specific method or task to perform the action. This

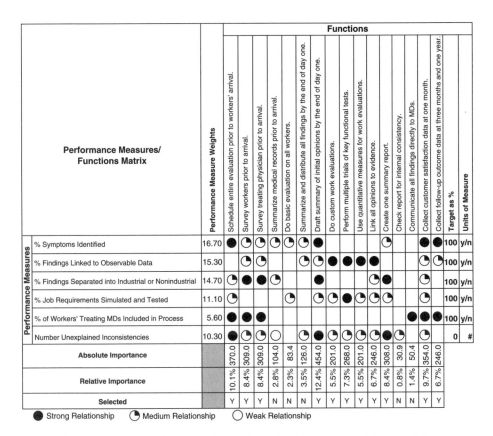

Figure 9.1. Performance Measures/Functions Matrix. This matrix translates performance measures into functions necessary to satisfy the customer. The importance of performance measures is used to identify important functions.

Source: Figure and calculations done with software from QualiSoft, 4652 Patrick Rd., West Bloomfield, Mich 48233, qualisoft@aol.com.

is what the service does, not its benefit. (Avoid verbs like *provide.*) The key functions are identified and become the columns of the matrix. Rows in function deployment can either be demanded qualities yielding a Demanded Qualities/Functions Matrix or performance measures yielding a Performance Measures/Functions Matrix.

In our example, the team used the Performance Measures/Functions Matrix (Figure 9.1). When the rows and columns were entered, the team looked at the relationships between functions (columns) and performance measures (rows). The strength of the relationship was decided by the answer to the question, "If this function exists, how much of an impact will it have on the performance measure?" The cells were then weighted, and the weighted importance of each was determined by adding the weights of the cells in the column and normalized by expressing the weight of each column as a percentage of the total weight of all columns (as in Step 2).

In this matrix, *Survey workers prior to arrival,* the second column under *Functions,* is a product of the highly weighted performance measures *% Findings Separated into Industrial or Nonindustrial* and *% of Workers' Treating MDs Included in the Process.*

EXERCISE 9.1

- Enter the Performance Measures (or Demanded Qualities) into the rows of a Performance Measures/Functions Matrix (or Demanded Qualities/Functions Matrix) (blank sample in Appendix A). Enter the weights of Performance Measures (Demanded Qualities) into columns.

- Enter the Primary Functions into the columns. These are the Primary Functions for the critical paths.

- Evaluate the relationship between the Performance Measures (Demanded Qualities) and Primary Functions by asking, "If you provided Function *A* (column), how necessary is it for Performance Measure *Y* (row)?"

- Rate these relationships as

●	Strong	9
◑	Medium	3
○	Weak	1
	None	0

- Rate each cell by multiplying the weight of the Performance Measure (Demanded Quality) determined from the previous matrix (Step 2) by the value of the relationship in the cell.

- Columns are summed and the weight of each column expressed as a percentage of the total sum of the columns, again as done with the previous matrix in Step 2 and shown as Figure 9.1.

- Select the highly weighted functions and set targets for performance. These will be carried to the next step.

SUGGESTIONS AND CAUTIONS

Again, we want to emphasize that the strategy is to identify primary functions, not all functions and not all tasks. In healthcare, much of the delivery of service is done by healthcare professionals whose ongoing assessments are important and are required to make adjustments in delivery of service toward an outcome. At the present time, the level of the industry as a service provider and the state of underlying clinical information systems in accomplishing this task are relatively primitive. It is just not practical, let alone possible, to attend to every detail when designing many clinical services. Rather, the emphasis is on identifying what is important (targets), identifying important performance measures (feedback), and primary functions (actions).

Consider an elderly woman who is admitted to an acute care hospital with pneumonia. While she is there, she is noted to be poorly nourished. When friends are contacted, it becomes clear that the patient had "not been taking very good care of herself" prior to this illness. She may have no family. In the course of her evaluation and treatment, it becomes clear that she has a short-term memory impairment and it is unlikely to be safe for her to return to her previous living arrangements. She is also found to be incontinent of urine. For most elderly patients, an unspoken demanded quality is to return home or, if not, at least to something close to home and not an institution. This person is a good candidate to go into a board and care facility where she might have her own room, her meals and laundry would be done for her, and she might have some supervision with necessary medications. In order to meet this demanded quality, she would need to be continent of her bladder. So, a key performance measure of the success of her treatment would be 100 percent continence of urine.

A function commonly employed to achieve this measure is a toileting program. Patients are taught to empty their bladders frequently in order to be continent and to not have accidents. So here, frequent toileting would be an important function to achieve the performance measure of 100 percent continence and to get her back to the community. *Frequent toileting* is going to the bathroom every 3 hours. The task of taking the person to the bathroom could be performed by a nurse, a certified nurse assistant, a therapist who may be working with her in her self-care activities or endurance, and so on. In this "project," the target is to get the person to a community level, a key performance measure is 100 percent continence of urine, and a function—her treatment or care plan—includes frequent toileting. Tasks within that function include setting up a schedule and determining responsibility for who, when, and so on. The number of times she is incontinent could be used as a feedback measure of how the treatment is going.

In deploying this treatment plan, it would not be efficient to attempt to structure the daily tasks of every person who may participate in achieving this function throughout the entire day. Rather, this can be left to the treatment team, allowing them to work out a plan at their level to achieve the measure. A task for the project, however, might include assigning one person on the team to assess progress on a daily basis.

If a set of Performance Measures was already defined such as with the JCAHO's ORYX™ initiative (www.jcaho.com) they could be the input into Step 3.

STOP AND REFLECT

The link between customer demands and organizational actions continues to emerge. We have now identified key functions as sets of actions necessary to generate the targets for the future state (RNA) and the measures that will evaluate progress toward the target.

What is important? The QFD process to this point has identified:

- Customer segments that are important (chapter 6)

- Which demanded qualities are important to customers in these segments (chapter 7)

- Priorities for meeting these demanded qualities (chapter 8)

- Measures we are going to use to determine whether our actions are reaching the targets and measures of target performance (chapter 8)

- Functions we need to perform to deliver demanded qualities or influence performance measures (chapter 9)

Chapter 10

Failure Modes and Root Cause Analysis

Upon completion of this chapter, you will be able to:

- Identify how the service is most likely to fail

- Increase the robustness and reliability of the service before deployment

- Have an overview of tools used for sentinel event and root cause analyses

FAILURE MODE ANALYSIS

Up to this point, QFD tools have focused on what is important. What are the demanded qualities, and how will we measure our system for delivering them? Now we need to address the challenge that results from our human nature—our tendency to focus on the immediate problem or task. It is here that reinforcing and inhibiting (balancing) feedback are key to optimizing the function of the overall system. Feedback loops can be designed into the service process to bring the influences of key elements from long-term targets and desired outcomes to the present as we perform current functions and tasks.

Actual failure modes for a redesign project or potential failure modes for a new service are identified by various tools in this chapter. These failure modes are then addressed in New Process Deployment, Step 5 of the QFD process. If you are redesigning an existing system, the identification of failure modes is the search for the root causes of breakdowns in the current system.

We will discuss several tools to identify and prevent failure modes. These tools include diagrams, tables, matrices, and trees. The fishbone cause-and-effect diagram (Figure 8.2) is a basic tool. A variety of relationship matrices can be used for failure mode analysis. These include the Demanded Qualities/Failure Mode Matrix, the Performance Measures/Failure Mode Matrix, and a Functions/Failure Mode Matrix. The case study used a Functions/Failure Mode Matrix. We will also present several more traditional root-cause-analysis tools. These will include simple tables (such as Solutions Tables), complex tables (such as Failure-Mode-and-Effects-Analysis [FMEA] Tables), and tree structures (such as Fault Tree Analysis and Management-Oversight-and-Risk-Tree [MORT] Analysis). In the root cause literature, there are a number of additional tools, which include change analysis, barrier analysis, and events-and-causal-factor

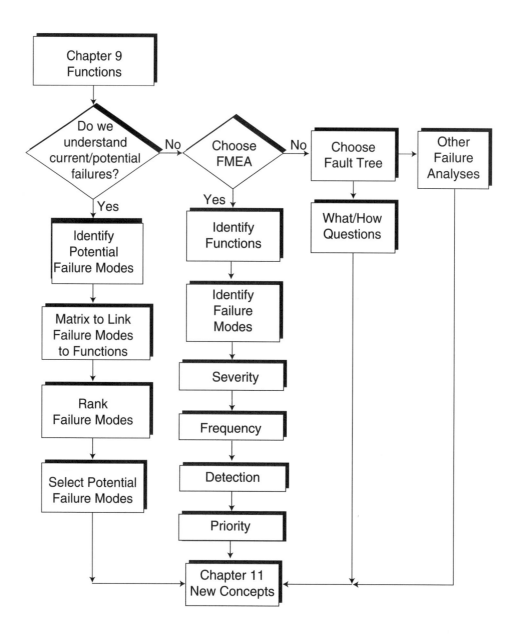

analysis, as well as those already mentioned. These additional tools will not be discussed here.

All of these tools will become commonplace in healthcare as the industry moves to meet the requirements of the Joint Commission on Accreditation of Healthcare Organizations' sentinel event policy. The Joint Commission is emphasizing the use of these tools to identify the root causes of breakdowns after they occur. Here, however, we are more interested in using them to design failure-proof systems. As healthcare matures as a customer-focused service delivery system, these tools will be used more and more frequently during system design to build reliability into services.

ROOT CAUSE ANALYSIS

Root cause is defined as the most basic reason for an undesirable condition or problem. When the root cause is eliminated, the undesirable effects do not happen. Root-Cause-Analysis methodologies identify causal factors.

The first step before embarking on the actual search in Root Cause Analysis is a high-level map of the process to be analyzed. The level of detail for the process map is decided upon, and the boundaries are set by the needs of the customer.

The next step is to define the problem or unwanted event. Only then does the team begin asking why the event occurred. Our first response to the question, "Why did (does) it break down?" is often not the true or root cause. First responses are usually symptoms or superficial elements—apparent causes in a longer causal chain (Figure 10.1). Symptoms must be distinguished from causes. In medicine, symptoms are seen as manifestations and are not the direct or root cause. This is also the case in root cause analysis. Patience and persistence are required to clearly distinguish between apparent causes and root causes.

Treating symptoms or apparent causes may give the appearance of improvement, but, if a more fundamental cause persists, then the problem will reappear. This is not to say that treating apparent causes has no value. The problem with treating apparent causes is that it reinforces the appearance of a problem with too many tasks and not enough resources. Root cause analysis and the tools described here allow the team to prioritize those potential failure modes or root causes that are likely to be most disruptive since designing solutions to these issues will have more value.

An organization's success with either failure mode prevention when designing new processes or deployment of solutions to root causes for existing problems is a function of:

1. The actual organizational commitment to the effort in practice versus spoken commitment

2. How carefully the analysis of current operations and processes is actually carried out during the analysis phase

3. The willingness to make needed changes, to install necessary controls and safety measures, to implement training, and so on

4. Whether the organization not only implements appropriate corrective and adaptive action but also takes the preventative actions that will preclude recurrence of unwanted conditions

A FAMILY OF FAILURE MODE MATRICES

We already presented examples where demanded qualities were mapped into performance measures and performance measures mapped into functions. Each one of these can be mapped into Failure Modes. There is value in all three of the mappings. Demanded qualities, performance measures, or functions are entered into the rows of a matrix. Then potential failure modes are identified by asking the question, "How and where could the processes break down if sabotaged by outside agents?" The common answer is the failure mode of the functions.

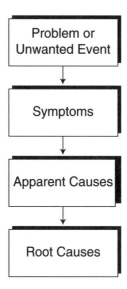

Figure 10.1. Root Cause Analysis. Root Cause Analysis begins with identifying the problem or unwanted event. Typically, symptoms and apparent causes are identified before identifying the underlying or root causes.

In the case study, a Functions/Failure Mode Matrix was used and primary functions were placed in the rows (Figure 10.2). The team used techniques such as brainstorming, data from the reliability column in the VOCT, past complaints, incident reports, and their collective past experience to identify likely breakdowns in service and modes of failure. If a large number of potential failure modes are identified, they can be organized by grouping techniques such as the affinity method and tree diagrams. The output is a ranking of the severity of the failure mode, but not its likelihood of occurrence. AHP can be used to rank the relative likelihood of occurrence. Assessments of relationships between columns and rows are made, cells weighted, columns summed, and so on, just as for previous matrices and as described in detail under Exercise 10.1.

EXERCISE 10.1

- Enter the key functions identified in Step 3 into the rows of the matrix and the percentage weight of function into the last column (Figure 10.2).

- Use brainstorming, data from the failure mode column of the VOCT, files of past complaints, incident reports, and past experiences to identify points where service has or could fail. Also, ask, "How and where could the process break down if sabotaged by 'outside agents'?"

- Determine the relationship between potential failure modes and functions by asking "If you knew that this breakdown or failure point occurred, how strongly would it affect the functions listed in the rows?"

Functions/Failure Mode Matrix	Weight of Functions	Incomplete evaluations, workers not completing requested activities	Having to add additional procedures and tests during evaluation period	Failure of team to adapt to unforeseen circumstances	Breakdown in team following policies and procedures	After evaluation period, discover some critical tasks are incomplete	Inconsistent findings between different physician evaluators
Schedule entire evaluation prior to workers' arrival.	10.1	●	◐		●		
Survey workers prior to arrival.	8.40	●		◐	◐		◐
Survey treating physician prior to arrival.	8.40		●	◐	◐		◐
Draft summary of initial opinions by the end of day one.	12.4		●	◐		◐	●
Do custom work evaluations.	5.50	●				◐	○
Perform multiple trials of key functional tests.	7.30					◐	○
Use quantitative measures for work evaluations.	5.50				◐	◐	
Link all opinions to evidence.	6.70					◐	◐
Create one summary report.	8.40		○				●
Collect customer-satisfaction data at one month.	9.70	●				●	●
Collect follow-up outcome data at three months and one year.	6.70					◐	
Absolute Importance		303	225	87.6	157	219	357
Relative Importance		22.4%	16.7%	6.5%	11.7%	16.2%	26.5%
Selected		Y	N	N	N	N	Y

● Strong Relationship   ◐ Medium Relationship   ○ Weak Relationship

Figure 10.2. Function/Failure Mode Matrix. This matrix is used to identify important failure modes for functions.

- To identify key potential failure points, weight the cells, sum the columns, and determine the percentage weight of each column, as done for matrices in Steps 2 and 3.
- Which are the most important failure modes?
- Use results in Step 5, New Process Deployment.

SOLUTIONS TABLES

A very simple failure mode or root-cause-analysis tool is called the Solutions Table (Figure 10.3). Solutions Tables have columns for the problems, the causes of the problems, the proposed solutions, and action. In the Solutions Table, the solutions identified should be solutions that will prevent recurrence of the problems.

For example, in Figure 10.3, two problems were identified when analyzing the cause of a patient fall. One was *Call light not used to call for assistance when needing to go to the bathroom.* Potential causes for this included *Patient(s) who is (are) Confused* and patients with *Urinary Incontinence and Urgency* who do not want to wait for help. A proposed solution would be *Frequent toileting of confused patients and patients with urinary frequency.* Actions would be *Staff education and feedback measures to monitor effectiveness.*

FAILURE-MODE-AND-EFFECTS-ANALYSIS (FMEA) TABLE

FMEA can be described as a systematized group of activities intended to:

1. Recognize and rank potential failures and effects of the failure on a product/process/service

2. Identify actions that could eliminate or reduce the chance of a potential failure occurring and/or improve detection

3. Document the process (*FMEA* 1995)

FMEA is a bottom-up systematic procedure. Its goal is to identify potential failure modes, assess and rank the effects of these upon the customer, identify potential causes, and identify methods for prevention or detection of failure conditions. FMEA can be used in the design stages of service or to analyze an already existing process or service. Ranking failures provides information to prioritize the use of an organization's limited resources. When completed, the table can be kept as a record. As high-ranking causes are eliminated, additional causes can be addressed.

FMEA analysis starts with functions, then considers failure modes and the effects of failure modes. The FMEA process also identifies the causes and severity of failures. The method of detection used and the effectiveness of detection methods are factors used to rank importance of the failure mode. Severity, Occurrence, and Effectiveness of Detection are combined into a composite score of criticality. This Risk-Priority-Number (RPN) score is used to rank the failure modes. The objective of FMEA is to minimize process failures and their effects on the process while also considering the needs and expectations of both providers and consumers. This information is placed in a table, as shown in Figure 10.4. Entries into the table follow the flow of the process.

Problem	Cause	Proposed Solution	Action
Call light not used to call for assistance when needing to go to the bathroom	Patient Confused Urinary Incontinence and Urgency	Frequent toileting of confused patients and patients with urinary frequency	Staff education and feedback measures to monitor effectiveness
Side rails not up	Patient was not assessed as fall risk. Staff did not follow Policies and Procedures.		

Figure 10.3. Solutions Table. A solutions table is a simple tool for recording the results of a root cause analysis. The table includes problem identification, cause identification, proposed solution, and action.

As a process, rehabilitation services can be mapped at a very high level (Figure 10.5). Potential patients are evaluated for admission (*Preadmission Screen*). If appropriate, they are admitted. They undergo an initial assessment to identify current capacities, future targets, and barriers. The patient's assets, strengths and weakness, for reaching the target are assessed. Failure or root cause analysis for this function is shown in Figure 10.4. A plan of treatment is developed (targets), actions are carried out (treatments), reassessments are made (measures), and the treatment plan is adjusted accordingly.

The preadmission assessment is carried out to determine if patients are appropriate for rehabilitation services. Information collected by this assessment is also used by the rehabilitation team as part of their initial evaluation and planning of care when the patient is unable to provide that information because of cognitive impairments due to stroke, brain injury, confusion, and so on, and family members or friends are not readily available. This preadmission assessment is also relied upon to capture the essential diagnoses made during the patient's stay in the acute hospital. Frequently, when patients are transferred from one hospital to another, the transfer records are incomplete. In one QFD project, a team was redesigning the core services of a rehabilitation hospital and a FMEA was carried out, as summarized in Figure 10.4. The columns of the table follow.

Function: the first column of the FMEA table lists the function of the step in the process to be analyzed. In this example, preadmission assessment and initial admission assessment are examples of function. The initial function of the process shown in Figure 10.5 is the preadmission assessment.

Potential Failure Mode: the next column is the potential failure mode, that is, how the failure would show up in the service. For this analysis, the team looked at how the failures would show up to the patient/customer and customer's family. For example, if the treatment team was not aware of a particular diagnosis, such as a patient with multiple trauma, the team would not understand why a patient was complaining of pain in the pelvic area because they would not know about the patient's fractured pelvis, and it would appear to the patient or family as confusion on the part of the team. Another patient might have had gastrointestinal bleeding and be losing blood into the gastrointestinal tract. If this data was not transmitted, testing for bleeding and anemia might not be done. This might show up as inaction by staff, an unmonitored condition, or failure to treat and protect the customer.

ITEM Function	Potential Failure Mode	Potential Effects of Failures	S E V	Potential Causes of Failure	O C C	Current Design Controls	D E T	R P N	Recommended Actions	Responsibility Target for Completion
Preadmission Assessment	Confusion on Part of Team	Less Available Resources	2	Inaccurate Data Missing Data Miscommunication Unnecessary Data	5 4 4 4	Informal "Gotcha" "Victim" Marketing Meeting	4	40		
		Wrong Treatment	4	Inaccurate Data Missing Data Miscommunication Unnecessary Data	5 4 4 4	Occurrence Reports Quality Concerns Chart Audits CM Survey	4	80		
		Missed Treatment (Unidentified Problem)	4	Inaccurate Data Missing Data Miscommunication Unnecessary Data Incomplete Tasks	5 4 4 4 5	Occurrence Reports Quality Concerns Chart Audits CM Survey	4	80		
		Rework		Inaccurate Data Missing Data Miscommunication Failed Expectations	4 4 4 2	Productivity Tracking	4	64		
	Condition Not Monitored	Missed Treatment (Unidentified Problem)	5	Inaccurate Data Missing Data Miscommunication Unnecessary Data	5 4 4 4	Occurrence Reports Quality Concerns Chart Audits CM Survey	4	100	Educate Staff in use of quality concerns and collect actual data.	2 Weeks, Clinical Department Managers
		Wrong Treatment	5	Inaccurate Data Missing Data Miscommunication Unnecessary Data	5 4 4 4	Occurrence Reports Quality Concerns Chart Audits CM Survey	4	100	Educate Staff in use of quality concerns and collect actual data.	2 Weeks, Clinical Department Managers
Initial Assessment on Admission										

Figure 10.4. Failure-Mode-and-Effects-Analysis Table. FMEA tables are used to recognize and rank potential failures and the effects of failures, to identify actions that could eliminate or reduce the chance of the failure recurring, and to document the process.

Potential Effects of Failures: this column lists examples of the effects of the failure on the system and on the end user, which here is the patient/customer. Examples listed in the figure include less available resources, wrong treatment, missed treatment, and so on.

Severity Rating (SEV): The team assesses the severity rating for each potential effect of the failure. In medical-device manufacturing, for example, there is substantial experience and a tradition of using severity ratings. There are a number of published scales for doing so. Severity rating scales for services, particularly in the delivery of healthcare, are not well developed.

As healthcare matures in the use of these tools, standard severity rating scores are likely to evolve. Severity scales may be different for an outpatient service, such as physical therapy, than for a service in the operating room or intensive care unit. The latter should parallel scales for medical devices such as defibrillators. The team in this study used the severity scale shown in the following text insert.

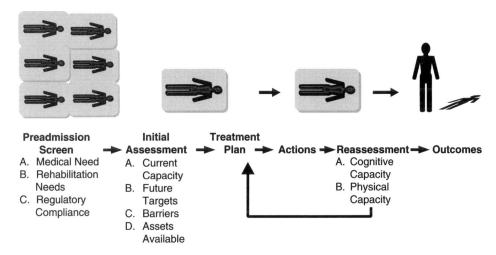

Figure 10.5. Inpatient rehabilitation as a process. The service line can be seen as a series of assessments and actions (treatments), followed by reassessments and adjustment of actions to produce desired outcomes.

Severity

1. Minor: almost no effect on the service or customer
2. Reduced service performance: undetected by the customer and no rework
3. Reduced productivity: service provider aware of the problem but customer is not, some rework
4. Minor adverse outcome but correctable: customer aware of the problem, can and needs to be fixed now, or leads to dissatisfaction
5. Potential for severe or major adverse outcome, with or without permanent consequences: customer detectable with much dissatisfaction, potential for no repeat business

---

For the potential effect of failure, *Less available resources,* the team assessed the severity rating as a 2, *Reduced service performance.* In contrast, for *Missed treatment,* such as internal gastrointestinal bleeding, the team rated the severity as 5, *Potential for severe or major adverse outcome, with or without permanent consequences.*

When rating severity, many healthcare professionals get trapped in "chaining." For example, a line could become contaminated during dialysis and the patient become infected. An infected person might not be appropriately treated and could become septic. A septic person who is not rapidly treated could go into shock. A person in septic shock could die. Death results not from that particular event of a contaminated line but from a series or chain of failures. When rating severity in the FMEA table, the severity is rated for the particular effect, not the overall result of a series of efforts.

*Potential Causes of Failure: t*he next column in the table lists the potential causes for each failure. Potential causes for *Condition Not Monitored* in the table included inaccurate data, missing data, miscommunication, and unnecessary data (i.e., too much data overwhelming viewer).

Occurrence Ratings (OCC): the next column in the table is an assessment of the probability of occurrence of a potential cause. The comments already made about lack of standard severity ratings for most hospital services are applicable here as well. Based on experience and ongoing quality activities, the team for the example in Figure 10.4 used frequency ratings shown in the following text insert.

Frequency	
1. < 1/100	Or, < two times/year
2. > 1/100 < 1/25	Or, < once/month and > 2 times/year
3. > 1/25 < 1/10	Or, < once/week and > once/month
4. > 1/100 < 1/5	Or, < once/day, but > once/week
5. > 1/5	Or, daily or multiple times/day

The team assessed the potential cause of failure of accurate data as 5, something that occurred multiple times per day.

Current Design Controls: this column lists current mechanisms in place that ensure that a potential failure does not arise or the procedures to detect a potential failure if it should happen. In this example, the team realized there were no formal processes or controls to address potential effects of the failures *Inaccurate Data* and *Missing Data,* which could lead to less Available Resources. The mechanisms that were present were informal and tended to be of a "gotcha" (a staff member from one department showing up how another department was not doing its job) or "victim" nature ("It's not my fault, because . . ."). On the other hand, for a *Wrong Treatment or Condition Not Monitored,* the organization had formal failure control structures in place, such as Quality Concerns and Occurrence Reports, Chart Audits, and Case Management Surveys.

Historically, occurrence or incident reports came into use to identify adverse outcomes. In the example organization, they had come to be used not only for detection and attempts at addressing system problems but also for identifying people problems that frequently resulted in "counseling." The staff tended to see incident reports as punitive and tattling. For this reason, the organization chose to use the quality concern as an internal way of capturing data for frequency.

Detection Rating (DET): for each design control, the effectiveness of the procedure is rated. As with severity and frequency, we are not aware of well-tested detection scoring mechanisms for healthcare services. The team in this example used the detection ranking shown in the following text insert.

Detection Ranking	
1. Remote/Almost impossible	Undetectable until catastrophe occurs
2. Very slight	Detectable by customer during service
3. Low–medium	Detectable before customer is aware
4. Moderately high–high	Detectable after the service is performed
5. Very high/Almost certain	Detectable before part of the service is delivered

Risk Priority Number (RPN): the RPN ranks the overall potential effect on patients and families and sets priorities for which to work on first. For the importance of each potential effect of a failure, a risk priority number is calculated by multiplying the severity rating by the occurrence ranking and the detection ranking.

$$RPN = (SEV) \times (OCC) \times (DET)$$

For the potential effect *Less Available Resources,* the severity rating was 2, inaccurate data occurred with a frequency of 5, and the detection method was very informal and rated as 4.

$$RPN = 2 \times 5 \times 4 = 40$$

In contrast, *Condition Not Monitored* had a severity of 5, an occurrence ranking of 5, and a detection ranking of 4.

$$5 \times 5 \times 4 = 100$$

The RPN for the effect is the highest product for severity, occurrence, and detection for that row of the table. This number is entered in the RPN column. Since the risk priority number is used for ranking, the team in the example would focus on eliminating the cause or designing a solution for eliminating *Condition Not Monitored* before *Less Available Resources.* Note: You may consider how this document would be used in a lawsuit.

In more mature industries, particularly in the medical-device industry, 10-point scales are used for severity occurrence and detection; hence, a wider distribution ranking is obtained. For teams working with this tool for the first time, if a standardized ranking for severity occurrence and detection is not available, we recommend using a five-point scale until the organization becomes familiar with the process. This reduces the amount of debate over the actual numbers. The hierarchical ranking is more important than the actual numbers. Ideally, an organization would work to eliminate all potential causes of failures. However, resources are not unlimited. This table is used to rank which failure modes should be worked on first. The important aspect of the process is not the number but the consistencies in rank. Scales for this tool will mature for the healthcare and other service industries as more data become available. The RPNs can be ranked in Pareto fashion. In practice, regardless of the resultant RPN, special attention should be given when the severity is high.

Recommended Actions: the next column lists recommended actions. A recommended action based on the results of the FMEA analysis was to redesign the form. This new form did not include extraneous data. This allowed people collecting the data to focus on critical information.

Responsibility: the next column identifies who is going to carry out the recommended action. A target date is entered into the last column (Figure 10.4).

Some organizations will add columns for severity rating, occurrence ranking, and detection ranking and calculate an RPN for what they expect after the recommended actions have been put in place. In general, the detection methods in health services for potential failures outside critical areas (lab, operating room, etc.) are relatively insensitive compared to those for manufacturing, Most manufacturing processes use a 10-point scale to improve likelihood of detection (Figure 10.6). Estimates of the effectiveness of such methods are shown in Figure 10.7. You will notice that in other settings, the detection methods routinely used in hospital settings such as policies and procedures (*Documented Work Instructions*) are not effective and chart audits (retrospective *Lot Sampling*) are only moderately effective, at best. This should not be surprising, based on the discussion of our biology presented in chapter 2.

EXERCISE 10.2

Follow the 16 FMEA steps to continue your exercises.

Steps for FMEA

1. Define the process.
2. Assemble data, information, and so on.
3. Draw a high-level block diagram of the process.
4. List the process items/functions that are going to be analyzed.
5. List the potential failure modes for each function.
6. List the potential effects for each failure mode.
7. Determine a severity rating for each effect.
8. Annotate any critical characteristics that may require additional process controls.
9. List all potential causes for failure mode.
10. Determine an occurrence rating for each potential cause.
11. List current process controls designed to ensure process adequacy.
12. Determine the detection rating for each potential cause.
13. Calculate a risk priority number (RPN) for each failure mode.
14. Determine recommended actions.
15. Assign responsibility and establish target dates.
16. Follow up.

Index	Effect	Subjective
10	Almost Impossible	Detection/mitigation is ineffective.
9	Remote	
8	Very Slight	Detection/mitigation is weak.
7	Slight	
6	Low	Detection/mitigation is moderately effective.
5	Medium	
4	Moderately High	Detection/mitigation is highly effective.
3	High	
2	Very High	Causes(s) cannot be expected to happen.
1	Almost Certain	

Figure 10.6. An example of a Manufacturing Detection Scale for the likelihood of detecting or improving process inadequacy. 10 is almost impossible to detect and 1 is almost certain to detect.

Stategy	Detection Rank
Testing	
100% with Automatic Removal	1–2
100% Manual with Removal	2–6
Lot-Sampling Techniques	4–6
First Articles	6–9
Inspection	
100% with Automatic Removal	1–2
100% Manual with Removal	2–4
Lot-Sampling Techniques	4–6
Form/Fit/Function	6–9
SPC Charts	4–5
Preventive Maintenance	3–9
Documented Work Instructions	7–10
Proactive Maintenance	2–4

Figure 10.7. Effectiveness of inspection strategies. This figure takes the index shown in Figure 10.6 and compares the effectiveness of the various strategies for inspection and ensuring quality.

FAULT TREE ANALYSIS

Fault Tree Analysis was developed initially in the Bell System, then modified and popularized in aviation by Boeing. Fault tree analysis is a top-down process. Root cause analysis begins with the identification of the failure. In QFD, it can begin with data from the VOCT2 in the failure mode column, complaints, incident reports, team experience, competitive benchmarking data, or the industry's literature. The list of basic symbols and definitions used in Fault Tree Analysis is given in Figure 10.8.

Figure 10.9 shows an example of Fault Tree Analysis for a patient who falls out of bed. The event was that the patient fell out of bed. Moving from top down, this could occur as a result of not having the side rails up *or* the patient's not using the call light for help with getting to the bathroom, then getting up and falling.

At the next level, the side rails may not have been up because the patient was not identified as a fall risk *or* staff did not follow through with appropriate policies and procedures if the patient was identified as a fall risk. The call light may not have been used because the patient was both confused *and* having urinary incontinence and frequency and did not want to wait for help. This visual way of showing the system structure and the relationships between events facilitates identifying corrective action.

Estimates can be used to rank the probability (P) of occurrence of events within the table:

- For AND gates, the probability equals P (A) × P (B).

- The probability for an OR gate can be approximated by adding
  P (A) + P (B) − P (A > B).

The team focuses on high likelihoods and common causes to identify solutions. Solutions usually involve reducing a particularly long series of events required to prevent occurrence or building redundancy into the system to prevent the occurrence. A strategy for identifying solutions to the Fault Tree is to add AND gates to the process so that the probability of occurrence is reduced.

EXERCISE 10.3

Continue Exercise 10.2 by identifying AND and OR gates.

MANAGEMENT-OVERSIGHT-AND-RISK-TREE (MORT) ANALYSIS

Management-Oversight-and-Risk-Tree Analysis was developed by the Department of Energy. It is a tree diagram that begins with the top event, which is the accident or incident under investigation. At the second level, as the name implies, the tree includes both management oversight and assumed risk.

The basic premise in the MORT analysis is that any accident is due to either Management Oversights and/or Omissions or an improperly Assumed Risk. In Figure 10.10, *Fall with Injury* is the event (Level 1). Level 2 of the figure illustrates that this could occur as the result of *Management Oversights and Omissions and/or Assumed Risk.* In a rehabilitation hospital, for example, the goal is to promote independence, so mobile patients with minimal restraints are desirable. However, these conditions are accompanied by the assumption of some risk. Falls with injuries could occur either from omissions or assumption of too much risk.

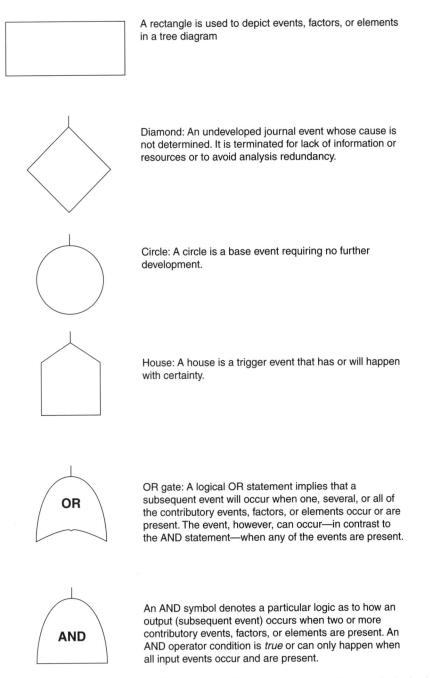

A rectangle is used to depict events, factors, or elements in a tree diagram

Diamond: An undeveloped journal event whose cause is not determined. It is terminated for lack of information or resources or to avoid analysis redundancy.

Circle: A circle is a base event requiring no further development.

House: A house is a trigger event that has or will happen with certainty.

OR gate: A logical OR statement implies that a subsequent event will occur when one, several, or all of the contributory events, factors, or elements occur or are present. The event, however, can occur—in contrast to the AND statement—when any of the events are present.

An AND symbol denotes a particular logic as to how an output (subsequent event) occurs when two or more contributory events, factors, or elements are present. An AND operator condition is *true* or can only happen when all input events occur and are present.

Figure 10.8. Fault tree symbols. This figure lists commonly used symbols in fault tree analysis.

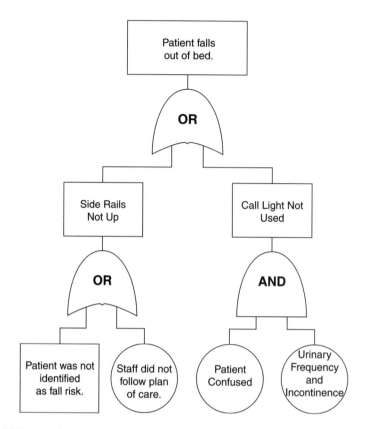

Figure 10.9. Fault Tree Analysis. The event was a patient falling out of bed. Potential causes for the event are outlined in the tree.

Level 3 of the tree shows that *Management Oversights and Omissions* could result from oversights or *Omissions in Management System Factors or Specific Control Factors.* At Level 4, management systems might be defined as *Policies, Implementation or Risk Assessment Systems.* A fishbone diagram can be used to fill out the list of potential causes for failure at these lower levels of the tree. For example, when *Amelioration* is placed at the head of the diagram, the lack of a way of alerting staff when an unsafe patient is getting up could be identified as a cause for falls. A solution could be corrected by an alarm. Specific control factors could include barriers and controls such as side rails on the bed and a lap belt when the patient is sitting in a wheelchair. Amelioration of specific causes could include adding a bed alarm that goes off when the patient attempts to get out of the bed, a wheelchair alarm when the patient attempts to get out of the wheelchair, and/or a lap belt when the patient is sitting in a wheelchair.

SUGGESTIONS AND CAUTIONS

The particular tool or tools used in Failure Mode Analysis should be determined in part by the type and location of the service being designed. For an outpatient service or service like the one in the example where consequences of failure are usually customer service rather than patient injury issues, a matrix or simple table may be adequate. For ser-

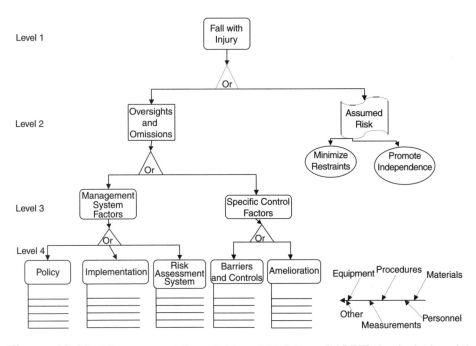

Figure 10.10. Management-Oversight-and-Risk-Tree (MORT) Analysis. Level 1 is the event. Level 2 contrasts oversights and omissions versus assumed risks. Level 3 looks at management system factors and specific control factors, a breakdown of which might lead to such an event. Level 4 looks at specific factors that contribute to these.

vices that may potentially result in severe patient injury (e.g., use of a device in an operating room), more detailed tools might be more appropriate, such as FMEA or Fault Tree Analysis, which include estimations of probabilities of occurrence, severity, and detection. The team should not use multiple tools during the design process but should pick the tool that seems to best fit the service being designed.

For some services, failure deployment might be more appropriately carried out after key concepts have been selected for the service through development of the process map, that is, after new process deployment (Step 5). For some services, Steps 4 and 5 are alternately revisited in order to enhance the efficiency and reliability of the service. Again, how much time and detail the team spends at this level of the QFD process should depend upon consequences of failure and the maturity and competitiveness of the environment for the service being rendered. QFD has a variety of tools. The team decides where to start and picks the best tool. When the output of that tool is understood, the team is positioned to select the next most appropriate tool.

STOP AND REFLECT

You now have revealed potential failure modes and given the team the opportunity to design a more robust service system.

Chapter 11

Creating and Selecting Concepts for Service Delivery

Upon completing this chapter, you will be able to:

- Evaluate alternative designs
- Generate new concepts

I f the current process is inadequate to perform a key function or deliver a performance measure target level, it is necessary to develop new processes to perform these
functions. In some cases, these may be entirely new processes. In other cases,
change with subprocesses or steps within subprocesses will be sufficient to address the
inadequacy.

In this step, the team will construct high-level flowcharts, design processes, and
subprocesses to deliver key functions and performance measures, then select between
alternatives. Rather than being a series of linear steps, this process is often a reverbera-
tion between designing a process, developing a process flowchart, and making process
selections. This interplay is managed by tools that continuously focus the QFD team on
what is important.

Since our social organizations are extensions of our biology, the same fundamental
structures that underlie cell function are replicated in our bodies and our social networks. As in the cell, changes in organizational behavior require clear targets and critical feedback. Often, efforts to change or redesign a process do not incorporate feedback
that links organizational performance to the target (demanded qualities); nor do they
provide critical feedback to determine whether the organization is meeting the targets.
Relying exclusively on narrowly focused feedback measures such as volume and dollar
revenue is insufficient in today's world.

Just as with earlier steps in the QFD process where the team was faced with multiple demanded qualities, multiple performance measures, and multiple functions or multiple failure points, teams often generate multiple concepts for the various functions in
the service. Keeping the team focused on what is important, selecting concepts that
account for and build in reliability, and incorporating balancing and reinforcing feedback at key steps in the process are critical to successfully shifting an organization's

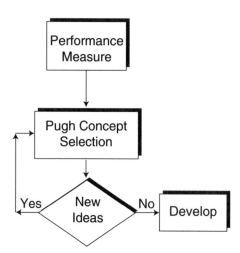

behavior. The tools for choosing concepts can be as simple as AHP pairwise comparisons between multiple concepts or as detailed as a Concept Selection Matrix.

NEW PROCESS DEPLOYMENT

To illustrate key parts of New Process Deployment, we present two partial examples. In Step 3 of the case study, *Create one summary report* was identified as a key function. In the Functions/Failure Mode Matrix of Step 4, *Inconsistent findings between different physician evaluators* was identified as a highly weighted potential failure mode.

When designing the concept from the perspective of a failure mode, incorporating reinforcing (positive) or balancing (negative/inhibiting) feedback to ensure optimal output for a function is one strategy to prevent the failure mode. Another is to incorporate barriers that prevent its occurrence.

The process of concept selection and generation developed by Stewart Pugh will be used to rank alternative concepts (Pugh 1991). The Pugh process was initially developed to make paired comparisons between the provider's "product" and the industry's current best. Several criteria are used and may be weighted. New designs are developed by integrating the best features onto a common platform.

The team generated three concepts for performing this function in a way that would reduce potential inconsistencies in the report. Each concept included a feedback loop to shape consistency between evaluators in the final report (Figure 11.1). The concepts involved a series of phone calls, a series of faxes, or a face-to-face meeting between all physicians. Constraints such as organizational time, cycle time, costs, and consistency were chosen as dimensions to evaluate strengths and weaknesses of each of these potential options.

First, the team used the AHP process to weight these four constraints. The four constraints and their weightings were then placed into the rows of the New Concepts Matrix (Figure 11.1). The competing concepts were placed in the columns. Each concept is shown as a flowchart. In practice, the flowcharts are often on the wall and labeled as A, B, C or 1, 2, 3. To select the best concept between the alternative designs, one concept is chosen as a reference. In this example, Concept 2 was chosen as the reference. With this reference point, each of the four constraints for the remaining two concepts are

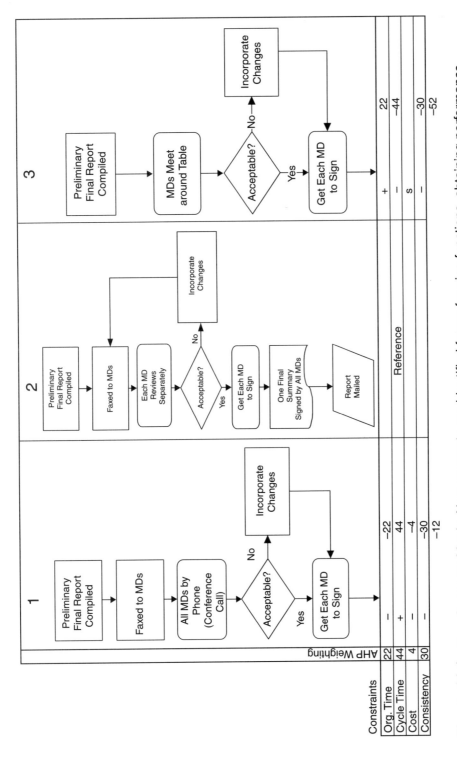

Figure 11.1. New Concepts Matrix. New concepts are identified for performing functions, obtaining performance measures, or delivering demanded qualities. Competing functions are ranked based on weighted criteria, and the most heavily weighted concepts are selected.

compared as either + (better), S (same), or - (worse) than the reference concept. These values are placed in the appropriate cell.

As in our other matrices, the cells are then weighted by multiplying the rating (+ equals 1, – equals –1, and S equals zero) times the AHP weight. The columns are then summed. In this particular example, the reference (Concept 2) rated higher than either Concept 1 (–12) or Concept 3 (–52). It was thus chosen as the design concept for this particular part of the overall service chain.

If the reference was not the best, the new best becomes the reference and the process of comparison is repeated. Once the reference concept has been established, incremental improvement of the reference is attempted. Looking at all the options, there may be some piece that is better in one of the nonselected options that can be incorporated into the reference concept. For example, Concept 3 is better for *Organization Time* and Concept 1 is better for *Cycle Time*. It is useful to explore whether the system components that create these better performances in the other concepts can be included in the reference concept.

VARIATION AND CUSTOMER SATISFACTION

The performance of a system is evaluated by measuring the average performance and the variation of performance (Figure 11.2). Consider the performance measure time to complete an evaluation, which is plotted on the horizontal axis. Customer satisfaction is plotted on the vertical axis (from high satisfaction at the base to dissatisfaction). Customer dissatisfaction increases with increasing time (upward sloping curve). Here, the shorter (smaller) the time, the better (smaller is better), as shown in the figure.

When comparing systems, if two systems, System A and System B, have the same average but different variations, the system with the smaller variation would be better (Figure 11.3). If the two systems have the same variation but different averages, the one with the lowest average time to complete the evaluation would yield more customer satisfaction and hence be more desirable (Figure 11.4).

Figure 11.5 depicts two systems, one with a lower average but more variation, the other with a higher average but less variation. Here, on average, System B will be lower in time but System A will be more consistent. What do you do if both the average and the variation are different? Use Taguchi's Loss Function (see Appendix C and Terninko 1989).

EVOLUTION OF SYSTEMS

Biologists have reflected back over time and identified patterns of change that have occurred in various species and living systems. Similarly, the Russian scientist Genrich Altshuller looked for and identified patterns in the evolution of technical systems (designed by humans). Terninko, Zusman and Zlotiv, 1998 identified eight principles that underlie the direction of evolution in technical systems:

1. Stages of evolution of a technological system (evolution along an S curve)

2. Evolution toward increased ideality

3. Nonuniform development of system elements

4. Evolution toward increased dynamism and controllability

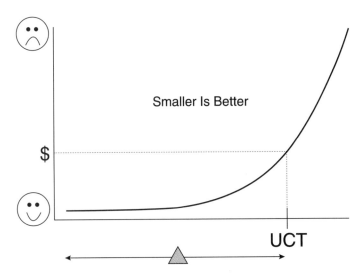

Figure 11.2. Variation and customer satisfaction in performance. Smaller is better. The performance of a system can be evaluated by measuring its average performance variation. Here, the performance measure is the time to complete an evaluation. Customer satisfaction would increase with decreasing time.

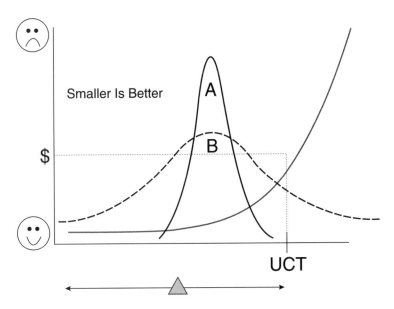

Figure 11.3. Smaller variation is better. Customer satisfaction (very satisfied at the bottom and very dissatisfied at the top) is plotted on the vertical axis, and performance measure is plotted on the horizontal axis. The performance of a system is evaluated by measuring not only average performance but also the variation of performance. Systems A and B have the same average with different variation. The system with the smaller variation would be the better.

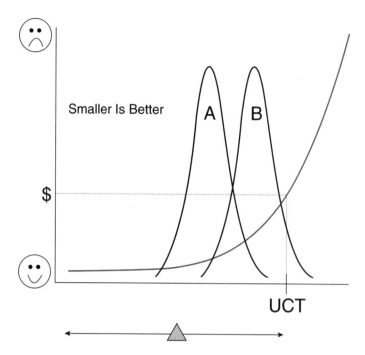

Figure 11.4. Smaller average is better. Customer satisfaction (very satisfied at the bottom and very dissatisfied at the top) is plotted on the vertical axis, and performance measure is plotted on the horizontal axis. If two systems had the same variation but different averages, the one with the lowest average time to complete the evaluation would be more desirable.

 5. Increased complexity followed by simplification

 6. Evolution with matching and mismatching elements

 7. Evolution toward microlevels and increased use of fields

 8. Evolution toward decreased human involvement

These observations indicate that there are only eight major directions in which systems evolve. For example, consider Pattern 8, *Evolution toward decreased human involvement.* Diagnostic functions that were once done by physicians are now done by technical systems, such as CAT scans, MRIs, and laboratory chemistries. In the future, other functions now carried out by physicians will be done by technical or mechanical systems such as diagnostic and treatment algorithms and decision support software. *Nonuniform development of system elements* is another example. Most people in healthcare embrace the introduction of the information technology infrastructure. They see it as facilitating access to data, reports, and so on in a more timely manner. But many, for example physicians, resist the use of this technology by managed care companies to deliver care with less variation.

Not every component of a system has the same level of performance. The weakest link in a chain is where the effort for improvement should be made. We often have a component of a system that is our favorite to improve, even when it is not the bottleneck. To spend resources on a component because it is our *favorite* when it is not the weak point in this system is not the best use of limited resources.

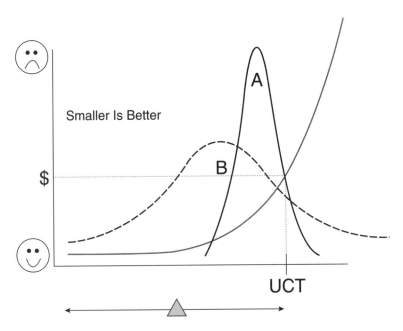

Figure 11.5. Which is better? Customer satisfaction (very satisfied at the bottom and very dissatisfied at the top) is plotted on the vertical axis, and performance measure is plotted on the horizontal axis. If both the average and the variation are different, use the Taguchi Loss Function.

Not reflected in the patterns of evolution is the notion that everything has a positive and a negative aspect. It is important to identify both of these aspects and minimize the negative. More detail on the eight patterns of evolution is available in Appendix D.

THE IMPORTANCE OF REINFORCING (POSITIVE) AND BALANCING (NEGATIVE) FEEDBACK

At its core, healthcare as a delivery system is a series of chain handoffs that creates value for customers. Chain handoffs require the coordination of actions between people. The efficiency of the chain handoff processes can be increased by shortening their length, increasing their throughput, or decreasing variations across the handoffs. In healthcare, like many service industries, the most common points of failure in the process are breakdowns in the management of commitments—a breakdown in the Action Workflow Cycle (Figure 3.7). Many times when healthcare workers expect something and it is not done, say to receive a report, they examine where the breakdown occurred and find that:

1. The customer did not clearly spell out the conditions to satisfy his or her request (I want a, b, c by time Y).

2. The provider did not clearly understand the conditions of satisfaction.

3. The provider did understand but failed to keep the commitment.

4. Unforeseen circumstances arose, and the provider failed to renegotiate the promise with the customer.

Let us revisit the example where our case study organization was asked to generate reports in a more timely manner. When the steps that generated the final report were mapped out, the biggest delays were in getting the most highly trained professionals, that is, the physicians, to submit their reports. Physicians are a major source of variation in healthcare. A major portion of the struggles in "managing care" and building quality and efficiency into a healthcare center is reducing variation in physician behaviors.

This segment of the process was mapped out as shown in the flowchart (Figure 11.6A). Using the basic cycle for the exchange of value between humans (i.e., the cycle of human commitment as previously presented in Figure 3.7), a process map was developed (Figure 11.6B). We made a claim earlier that systems function in perfect alignment with their underlying structure and sets of relationships. The organization continued to send patients to the physicians even though it was not satisfied with the timeliness of reports. This action rewarded and reinforced less-than-desirable behavior.

When the team examined the breakdown in getting timely reports using the workflow model, it became clear that they had not clearly defined and negotiated a specific due date with all the physician providers. Instead, the expectations were a nebulous "as soon as possible." (These reports often become legal documents that undergo scrutiny and challenge, therefore requiring multiple edits on the part of the physician for clarity, consistency, and conciseness.)

Once the team identified this breakdown, they clarified and negotiated a definite time commitment for completion of the report by each physician—one week after completion of the evaluation. A new step to check that these conditions of satisfaction were met was added. If the conditions were not met, immediate feedback to the physician was generated by a phone call (Figure 11.6B). The new process could be mapped in standard flowcharting terminology (Figure 11.6C).

When this aspect of the process was deployed, an administrative person in the marketing office who managed the flow of reports was to check at one week after the injured worker had been discharged to see if all the reports had been received. If a report was missing, a call was placed to the physician, generating immediate feedback. If the report was still not received within several days, a second call was made by that same person. If the report still failed to arrive, a third call by the managing physician (physician peer) was made to ask if there was some way that the organization could assist that provider in meeting this deadline and future deadlines.

This feedback quickly modified behavior, clarified commitments, and redesigned the process at this step, resulting in the reduction of total cycle time (Figure 4.11) for when the injured worker was discharged from the facility until the final report was in the hands of the insurer from a mean of 50 days to 18 days (Chaplin 1996). Both the average time and the variation for the system decreased.

A very robust strategy for designing feedback is creating feedback that stops the process from moving forward until certain conditions of satisfaction have been met. This is analogous to the example of the Toyota production system that empowered the line worker to stop the line if defects were identified. This strategy can also be incorporated into patient care.

In the following example, a rehabilitation hospital had relicensed one-half of their beds under a skilled nursing license and called itself a transitional rehabilitation unit. Federal regulations governing acute hospitals and skilled nursing facilities differ. In the skilled nursing facility, the use of sleep medications might be classified as chemical restraints.

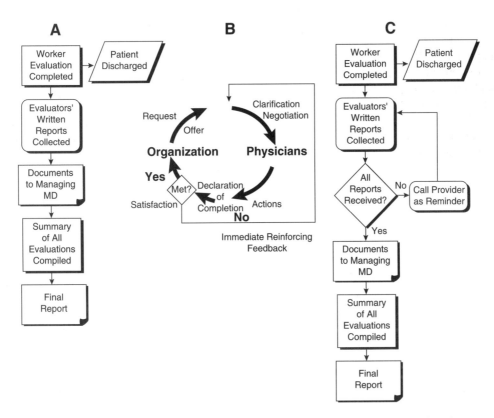

Figure 11.6. Importance of self-organizing feedback. The team has previously experienced delays in generating a final report. The root cause for these delays was a delay in getting consulting phyisican experts to submit their reports. This step was mapped out. Balancing feedback to stop the process and to generate immediate feedback to modify behavior was added.

Shortly after the new unit opened, concern arose that the pattern of ordering sleep medications, although judged medically appropriate, might be interpreted as a violation of these regulations. The regulations are operationally interpreted by surveyors in the field as requiring that nonmedication sleep measures, such as quiet and warm milk, first be exhausted before sedative hypnotics are used. Many people who enter skilled nursing facilities do so because they can no longer manage at home, and the skilled nursing facility will become their new home. These regulations were designed to protect this customer segment. Many such facilities in the community had adopted a strategy of not prescribing sedative hypnotic medications for a period of time after admission as a way to comply with the intent of the regulation. However, patients admitted from an acute hospital to the rehabilitation facility were often recovering from an acute illness or extensive surgery, had spent time in an intensive care unit, or were in pain and exhausted. For these people, three to four nights of restful sleep are extremely beneficial. Therefore, a decision was made to not adopt the strategy of withholding these medications.

Using the workflow model presented in Figure 3.7, the *as is* process has been mapped (Figure 11.7). By writing in the chart, a physician or nurse initiates a request.

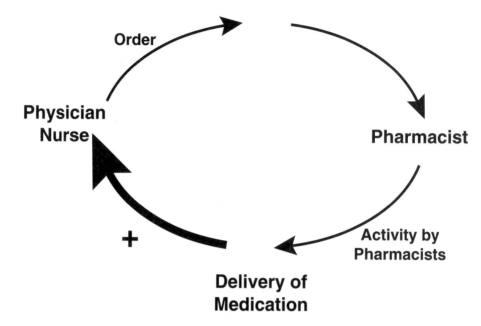

Figure 11.7. *As Is* Systems contain feedback. The action workflow for obtaining a sedative hypnotic is shown. The organization was reinforcing undesirable behavior by filling incomplete orders. Such activity was reinforcing the *as is* process.

Clarification may or may not be required. The pharmacist performs the actions needed to deliver the request (i.e., sleep medication) to the floor. These sleep medications were distributed, with the staff intending to complete the necessary documentation later. In this case, the delivery of the medication with absence of the appropriate documentation was reinforcing behavior that might be judged as noncompliant with regulations by outside surveyors at the risk of fines of $10,000/occurrence.

Faced with the problem of reducing this risk, the team in this example defined a set of conditions that were judged appropriate for the use of sedative hypnotics, as well as for minor tranquilizers. A set of conditions for satisfactorily documenting justification for the medication was also defined. The two sets were linked by requiring a completed written document before the medication could be dispensed. A one-page order form was designed as a tool to facilitate documentation. After review by the appropriate committees, the pharmacist was empowered to decline the request for a sedative hypnotic or minor tranquilizer if both sets of conditions were not satisfactorily met.

Empowering the pharmacist to decline the request and then requiring the pharmacist to immediately transmit the rejection of the request back to the nurse meant the physician and the nurse had to modify the initial request (Figure 11.8). The actions of the pharmacist stopped the process, provided immediate balancing (negative) feedback, and forced those making an inadequate request to do more work.

Within days, old habits began to change. Within a few weeks, the number of incomplete orders being received by the pharmacy declined dramatically, reducing the potential for regulatory infractions and the risk of fines. In addition, there was a marked decrease in the number of sedative hypnotics prescribed per 1000 patient days per

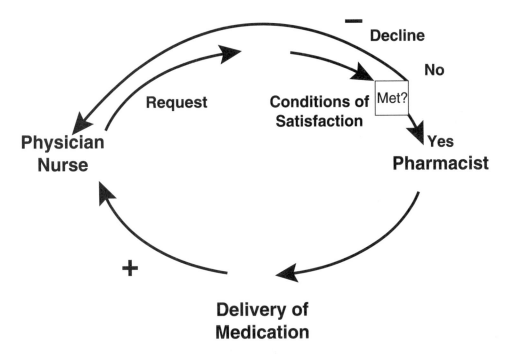

Figure 11.8. Importance of balancing or inhibiting feedback—a self-organizing process. Adding a specific and necessary data set of conditions of satisfaction empowered the pharmacist to decline to fill an order to stop the process if the conditions of satisfaction were not met. This created immediate negative feedback to the physicians and the nurse, requiring additional work.

month (Figure 11.9). Again, both the average and the variation about the average decreased. This resulted in reduced cost, as well as reduced exposure of patients to potential side effects such as residual drowsiness, balance problems, and falls (Chaplin et al. 1997).

EXERCISE 11.1

- Begin to draw a high-level flowchart for the functional steps in your overall process. For the purposes of this exercise, pick a function that has a strong relationship to a highly weighted failure mode identified in Step 4 with the functions/failure mode matrix (or the failure mode analysis tool you used).

- Generate high-level concepts to the design of this particular aspect of the process.

- Define a set of organizational constraints such as time, cost, and so on. For this exercise, choose at least three. If this is an actual process, define what your constraints in fact are.

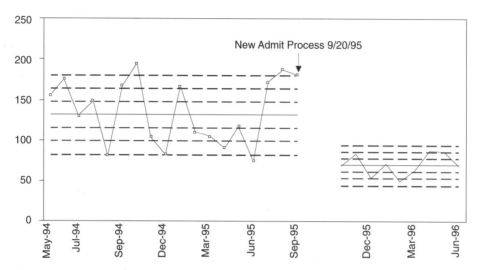

Figure 11.9. Sedative hypnotic use (rate/1000 patient days per month) results. Change in rate of dispensing sedative hypnotics after introducing balancing feedback. When balancing feedback was added, the use of sedative hypnotics substantially decreased, reducing costs and potential side effects to residents/patients.

Source: Ed Chaplin et al., *Quality Management in Healthcare* (Gaithersburg, Md.: Aspen Publishers, Inc., 1997). Used with permission.

- Use AHP to compare and weight these constraints and then enter the results into the rows of the New Concepts Matrix following the example in Figure 11.1.

- Enter the competing concepts into the columns.

- Choose one of the concepts as a reference point, and determine the relationship of each of the constraints with respect to this reference concept as + (better), S (same), or – (worse).

- Weight each cell by multiplying the AHP weight by the relationship rating.

- Sum the columns.

- Choose the most highly rated process.

- Create new concepts by integrating better subsystems from the other concepts.

- Reevaluate.

EXERCISE 11.2

Construct a high-level flowchart that links selected concepts for all key functions into an overall service process map.

SUGGESTIONS AND CAUTIONS

As with most steps in the QFD process, our embodied predisposition is to move rapidly to solutions and then jump into action and deployment. It is at this level, the introduction of reinforcing and/or balancing feedback around key functions, that we are able to overcome our human tendency to focus on individual components and short-term goals rather than the whole system and long-term goals. At the same time, this is an opportunity to build reliability, consistency, and reduced variation into our processes. The time invested here in identifying the key steps that most affect the mean output and variation in our process is well worth it.

Model studies of chaotic systems indicate that not all components within a system need to be regulated or controlled to stabilize the system. Rather, if reinforcing and balancing feedback is built into a key step, the system will self-organize into a stable form.

Also, when redesigning a process with QFD, remember to evaluate what aspects of the *as is* process have outgrown their usefulness and need to be discarded. Renewal and rejuvenation are journeys that include disintegration, discarding by-products, culling what is to be saved, realignment, growth, and reintegration. The seed germinates, and its actions grow a plant; the plant differentiates the flower, which matures into fruit, which embodies a new seed. The old plant dies, the seed germinates, and the species and life continue. Our physical bodies have efficient processes to catalyze change and renewal. Most of our current social organizations do not.

For example, our bodies have processes to discard what is no longer functional. During the fetal period, process structures and subsystems disintegrate when they are "outgrown." The bones of the hand develop within a single limb bud. The cells in the tissue between the future digits undergo a process called apoptosis (programmed cell death), which leads to the development of five separate digits. Again and again in nature we find models where what is valued is retained and what is a by-product or is no longer valued is culled out and eliminated as waste. Apoptosis and rejuvenation are key to balance and to the process of renewal and change. When you redesign a current system, remember to actively identify and discard tasks and measures that no longer add value.

STOP AND REFLECT

Concept design and feedback are the strategies to integrate differentiated parts, departments, people, and so on into the whole and to tie short-term actions to long-term results. By so doing, the future consequences of inadequate action are brought into the present.

This section introduces needed complexity, differentiating key steps, and concepts of functions within the whole. The differentiated actions remain linked and interconnected to the whole. The critical feedback that coordinates sets of relationships and connections with subsystems is given in more detail. This feedback will become differentiated targets (differentiated and local RNA) and feedback measures for the subgroups of people who will actually deliver the service within the larger process.

Chapter 12

Task Deployment

Upon completing this chapter, you will be able to:

- Determine which tasks are most critical to the new process

- Identify what equipment, space, tools, and training may be needed to catalyze the performance of these tasks

- Consider whether individual incentives—rewards, consequences, and performance criteria—need to be modified

The role of task deployment is to determine which tasks are most critical to the new process. Data comes from the process flowchart of the new process and from the performance measures and functions. The goal is for the team to determine what critical equipment and facilities (hardware), information systems (software), and human tasks (operators) are required for functions to be carried out, performance measures to be met, and self-regulating feedback to be created to ensure that demanded qualities have been delivered.

At this stage, the team can use either a Performance Measures/Task-Deployment Matrix or a Functions/Task-Deployment Matrix or go directly to the Task-Deployment Table. If the Performance Measures/Task or Functions/Task Matrices are used, the relationships between the Performance Measures or Functions rows and Task columns are determined. The tasks are weighted relative to each other, and targets for successful completion of the task are defined and incorporated into the Task-Deployment Table.

FUNCTION TREE

A function tree can be used for expanding the functions into tasks—going to the next level or levels—by asking a series of "what/how" questions. "What do we want to accomplish?" and "How are we to accomplish it?" The first level would be the function, and the next level would be the tasks associated with that function. Another level would define tasks at a greater level of detail (Figure 12.1). You continue this process of refinement until you know exactly what is necessary to satisfy the function. The relative importance of a task can be found by linking in a matrix.

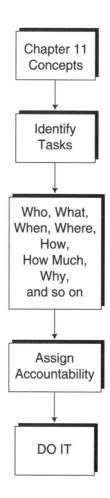

A function tree does not represent the actual linkages that exist between tasks and function. A hierarchy tree allows multiple connections between offspring and multiple parents (Figure 12.2). Using the Functions/Task Matrix is a convenient way to set the relative ranks for tasks based on their relationships to the functions.

Figure 12.3 shows part of the Function Tree from the case study. The function was to identify all capacities and impairments. To do this required knowledge of job functions. Calling the employer for job descriptions was identified as an important task in performing this function.

TASK-DEPLOYMENT TABLE

The typical Task-Deployment Table is similar to the example in Figure 12.4. Columns include:

- What (name of the task)

- Who (persons who will do it)

- When (time of day, week, month, frequency, etc.)

- Where (place, on site, off site, geography)

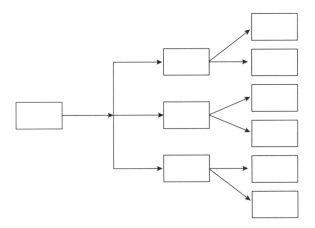

Figure 12.1. Hierarchy Tree 1. A function tree does not represent the actual linkages that exist between tasks and function.

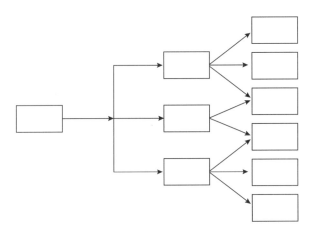

Figure 12.2. Hierarchy Tree 2. A hierarchy tree allows multiple connections between offspring and multiple parents.

- How (methods, tools, etc.)
- How much (it is here targets for the task would be entered)
- Why (reason the task is important to the customer, organization, etc.)
- Other (failure points, special skill requirements, training, education, etc., can be added here)

Types of tasks can also be separated and defined. For example, some tasks are critical to function, some tasks are critical to safety, and some tasks are critical to timing.

Upon completing task deployment, the team has already constructed a detailed picture of the overall target (demanded qualities), defined performance measures with measurable targets, and identified key functions and tasks required to meet these measures to ensure the

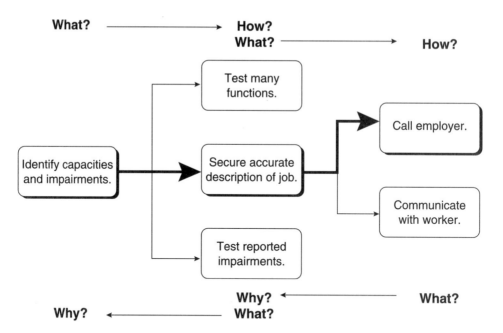

Figure 12.3. Functions Tree. Functional activity is necessary to achieve some target. Functions are identified and arranged into a hierarchy. In building such trees, if you start at a high level and move toward a lower level, you begin by asking the question "How?" In building the tree, if you move from a low level toward a high level, you ask the questions "Why?"

overall target to the process, that is, customer satisfaction, is being met. When you reach for an object, you are successful because you have by previous experience incorporated capacities to perform the necessary actions. At this level, a key question is, "Are human competencies and physical resources present and sufficient for the critical task and key functions in order to meet performance measure targets? If not, what is missing?"

EXERCISE 12.1

- Review the flowcharts for new concept designs, outputs from Performance Measures/Functions Matrices, and concepts for addressing failure modes in order to identify critical tasks.

- Place these tasks in the table, as shown in Figure 12.4.

- Determine who, what, when, where, and so on for the tasks.

- Determine if tools, training, additional space, job descriptions, skill requirements, and so on for the task are already present or need to be developed.

- Determine the who, what, when, where, and so on for training.

- Define a schedule for building competencies that are missing and introducing any needed tools and training.

What	Who	When	Where	How	How Much	Why	Other
All planning and preadmit scheduling is complete.	Marketing Secretary	Start 3 weeks prior to planned admit. Complete 5 days before	CRHSD	Phone and Fax		Build template for evaluation.	
Send and collect preadmit scheduling patient questionnaire.	Marketing Secretary	Send 2 weeks before planned admit.	CRHSD	Mail Phone		Build complete list of symptoms and impairments.	
Questionnaire sent and call made to treating physician.	Marketing Secretary Managing MD Peer to Peer	Survey 2 weeks. Call 1 week.	CRHSD	Mail Phone		Build complete list of symptoms, diagnoses, and impairments.	
Working summary completed at end of day 1.	Managing MD	Day 1.	CRHSD	Dictation		Get everyone on same page.	
First notification to evaluators when reports late	Marketing Secretary	Next working day after due date.	At MDs Office	Phone and Fax		Feedback to keep commitments.	
Third notification if report is late.	Managing Peer to peer	If misses deadline by 1 week or misses 3 deadlines in a row.	At MDs	Phone		Feedback to keep commitments or change commitments.	

Figure 12.4. Task-Deployment Table. Critical tasks are identified. The who, what, when, where, why, and how of the task are determined along with facility, equipment, any tools, and training that may be needed.

SUGGESTIONS AND CAUTIONS

Not every task needs to be put into the table. Sometimes all that needs to be provided is real-time reinforcing and balancing feedback to the team of professionals providing the service. Remember the discussion of the elderly woman in chapter 9. She was living alone prior to an episode of pneumonia, but, because of preexisting difficulties, the goal for her was to be discharged to a board-and-care facility in the community. The target for her treatment plan was to get her to a community level. A key performance measure was being continent of urine 100 percent of the time, and one of the functions in her treatment plan included being placed on the toilet every three hours. In deploying the treatment plan, it would not be efficient to attempt to structure the job of every person who may participate in achieving this function throughout the entire day. Rather, this can be left to the treatment team, allowing them to work out a plan at their level to achieve the measure. A task for the project, however, might include assigning one person on the team to assess progress on a daily basis and provide feedback to the rest of the team.

Professionals in healthcare services are very bright, goal oriented, and, by and large, overwhelmingly committed to doing what is right. Leaders and managers of a project team have the task of generating clear targets and good feedback in order to allow these professionals to be successful.

STOP AND REFLECT

This section sets targets and performance measures for key people within the process. It determines who receives the feedback. Despite common assertions of being customer focused, most healthcare organizations and their workers do what is easy and routine. To truly change a service, the change needs to occur at this "easy-and-routine" level (at the level of tasks).

Chapter 13

Closing the Loop: "Satisfaction Deployment"

Upon completing this chapter, you will be able to:

- Identify outcome measures for the process that relate back to the external environment (the customer)

- Explore ways this feedback will be disseminated through the organization to change not only individual, but collective, behavior

Cells continually capture data from the environment. Similarly, a robust and adaptable service must continually capture data from its customers. The *Plan, Do, Check, Act* (PDCA) cycle is a model for an adaptive system. Day-to-day operation will follow the *Standards, Do, Check, Act* (SDCA) cycle shown in chapter 5 until feedback indicates the system is not performing and shifts operation to the PDCA cycle. Any system design must have a PDCA cycle built in or else the system is at risk of slippage of its standards, and the organization will not become aware of the problem until failure occurs.

In our case study, three points from the process outlined in Figure 13.1 were chosen to evaluate outcomes from the customer's perspective (shaded numbers 1, 2, and 3 in figure). Data were collected at three months (Point 2) and one year (Point 3) postdelivery of service. Point 1 was defined as the time of determination that the injured worker had reached maximal medical improvement and was removed from the cycle of evaluation, treatment, and total temporary disability.

The organization reported follow-up data at three months and one year on 25 cases (Chaplin et al. 1999). At Point 1, 19 of the workers (76 percent) were determined to have received maximal medical treatment. For this group, residual impairments were defined and recommendations made with regard to vocational retraining. Further treatment was recommended for the remaining six workers (24 percent).

Follow-up data at three months indicated that, of the 19 cases for which a determination was made the injured worker had reached maximal medical improvement, the findings were immediately accepted by nine (47 percent) of the workers, their attorneys, and the insurer. The remaining 10 workers elected to enter into an appeal process. Follow-up

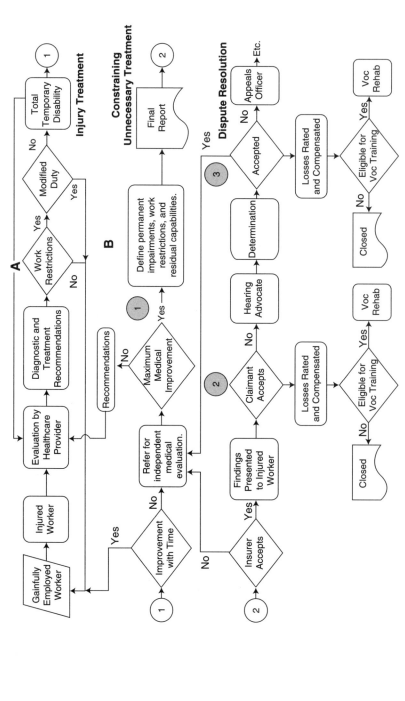

Figure 13.1. High Level View of Customer's Process. The first row focuses on a series of tasks and activities carried out for treating the acute injuries. The second row shows activities that constrain unnecessary treatment. A series of activities and tasks in the third row outlines activities for the dispute resolution. The organization in the case example provided tasks and functions shaded in the second row, labeled B. Details of this map are presented in a text box in Chapter 7. Three points within the process were chosen to evaluate outcomes from the customer's perspective (1, 2, and 3). Point 1 was defined by the time of determination that the injured worker had reached maximal medical improvement and was removed from the cycle of evaluation, treatment, and total temporary disability. Data were collected at three months (point 2) and one-year (point 3) post-delivery of service.

at one year indicated that three additional cases were settled without appeal, while two persons had appeal hearings in which the rulings upheld the completeness of the evaluation process and its accuracy, and the cases were closed. Two persons were still awaiting appeal hearings, one person died of a myocardial infarction unrelated to his work injury, and one case was lost to follow-up.

As presented earlier, over a five-year experience with this same customer base, the facility had averaged 22 ($\pm$4) evaluations per year (Figure 4.13). The QFD project started with interviews in the field in August of 1997, with implementation of the new system in November of 1997. Formal and informal feedback from customers since implementation was extremely positive. During 1998, the facility had evaluated 50 injured workers, a referral rate that is slightly more than double that of the average volume for past years.

EXERCISE 13.1

- Identify performance measures and collect data for the target outcome linking the process back to the external environment (the customer).

- Explain ways that the feedback can be disseminated throughout the organization to change individual behavior, as well as the collective behavior of the organization.

Figure 13.2 is a summary flowchart that gives an overview of the steps in QFD. More detailed flowcharts are located at the beginning of each chapter where the steps and tools are presented.

SUGGESTIONS AND CAUTIONS

Implicit in the task of reaching for an object and in our model of the cell as an organization is the principle that targets call forth action that is already embodied within the system (i.e., experiential knowledge, know-how). This action is modified by feedback about performance of functions aimed at achieving the target. All living systems, whether a simple flatworm in a pond or a human being in a social organization, can only change this embodied knowledge through new experiences, through actions. Old habits and ways of doing things are replaced by new learning. We learn through our interactions with the environment. In the absence of reinforcing and balancing feedback for new actions, our human tendency, particularly in the hurried mode of today's healthcare routine, is to default to old habits.

As shown through the experience with the sedative hypnotics in the skilled nursing facility (Figure 11.9), balancing feedback supplied at a critical step in a process can radically transform the outcome. It was not a conceptual knowledge deficit on the part of the staff that contributed to the sedative hypnotic problem. The process action team that was appointed to resolve the problem had gone to the staff, and the staff knew why it was important to adequately document the need for sedative hypnotics. They were aware of fines, regulatory requirements, and so on. But in the hectic day-to-day activity of caring for an increasingly larger number of patients with fewer people, the staff needed help in the form of inhibiting feedback to ensure that the process did not go forward until conditions of satisfaction were met.

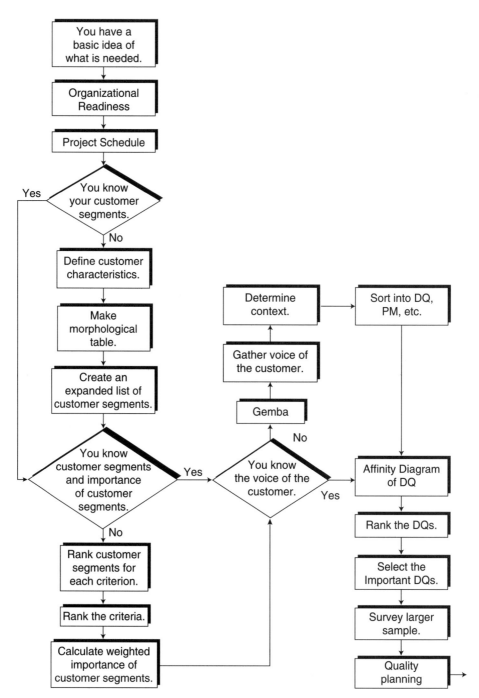

Figure 13.2. A sample flow chart of a comprehensive QFD process. This shows the flow for the case example. More detailed flow charts for each step are presented at the beginning of the chapters where these tools are initially presented and discussed. This is presented to give you, the reader, an overview review of the flow. As noted in the text in their respective chapters, which of the tools are used depends on the project and the nature of the organization's structure and function.

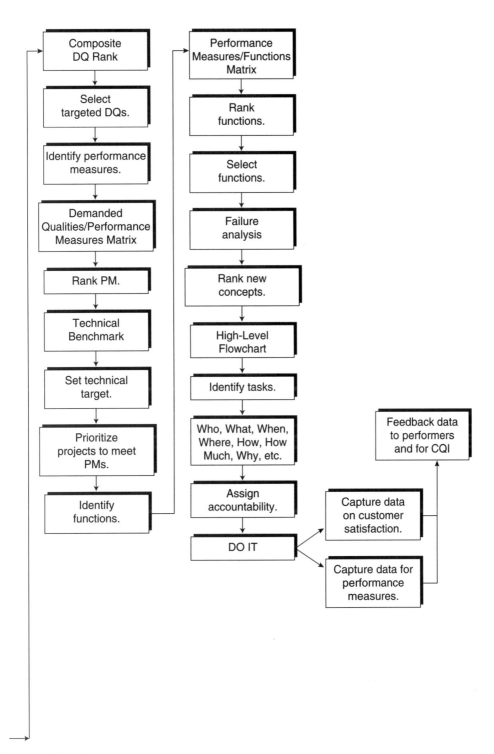

Figure 13.2. *Continued.*

For organizations as well as for individuals, change is more easily said than done. It takes weeks, months, and often a few years for fundamentally new processes to take hold and become the dominant practices of a culture. Just as feedback is critical to the cells in your body, the organization needs feedback from customers on how they are doing. A robust QFD process includes steps to capture ongoing feedback from customers to the organization and the people delivering the service.

The discussion presented in this chapter, closing the loop, is usually not part of classic QFD. Indeed, one of the prepublication reviewers suggested that we call the entire text Satisfaction Deployment, not Quality Deployment. We were not bold enough to do so but did take the suggestion and add it to the title of this chapter. Quality Function Deployment traditionally focuses on customer needs and performance measures of these needs. We, however, see customer satisfaction through the exchange of value between customer and organization as the lifeblood of any organization, hence the emphasis on closing the loop as a way for continuous quality improvement (CQI).

As shown in Appendix E, Figure E.9, the initial case example included the performance measures *Collect customer-satisfaction data at one month* and *Collect follow-up outcome data at three months and one year.* The first was included as a measure of customer satisfaction with the delivery of the service, the second as a measure of whether customer needs had been met and whether customers were and/or remained satisfied.

Will a robust QFD process eliminate all undesired variability in a service and always satisfy the customer? The answer to this question is, of course, *No.* QFD is a set of tools to generate a robust hypothesis for the whats and hows to accomplish that. Capturing data about the service's actual performance and customer satisfaction helps manage and continuously improve the service.

STOP AND REFLECT

In this section, we have closed the loop by providing customer feedback on organizational priorities to the organization's leadership, management, and service providers.

Chapter 14

Blitz QFD

Upon completing this chapter, you will be able to:

- Identify the critical few Performance Measures, Functions, Failure Modes, and Tasks
- Have an upwardly compatible start for Comprehensive QFD

Many organizations initially see the comprehensive nature of QFD as too demanding of resources, or they are in a hurry to get started with significant improvement for current design processes. Some organizations and consultants overcome this inertia by using what has been coined *Blitz QFD* (Zultner, 1998). Here, the number of items addressed at each step (after capturing the voice of the customer) is reduced, but the characteristics of the steps themselves are not diminished.

Blitz QFD, like comprehensive QFD, starts with identifying customer segmentation, prioritizing and gathering the voice of the customer, and selecting a relatively small number of demanded qualities. Unfortunately, these first steps in the QFD process cannot be compromised. If you use the voice of your organization for identifying the few important demanded qualities, you will not develop a customer-driven system. You would be making the same mistake as Michael Dell, president of Dell Computers, when the company developed a new line of equipment based on their excitement for the technology (Dell and Fredman 1999). After hiring a large number of talented people to design the Olympic family of products, they got the following reaction at the COMDEX trade show, "Thanks very much but we don't need that much technology." They had developed a line of product for themselves instead of for the customer.

Recall that the goal of the QFD process is to link the organization to its customers to enhance the exchange of value (Figure 14.1):

- The process begins by identifying customer segments that are important to the organization (Figure 14.2).

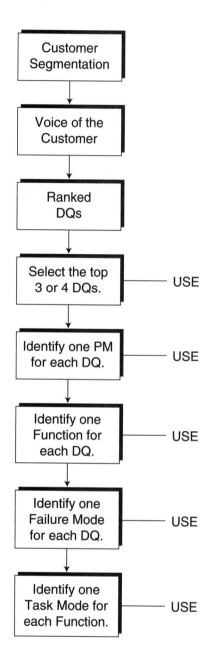

- The team then works with customers to identify and rank customer needs and wants as demanded qualities (Figure 14.2). The demanded qualities the organization will focus on to satisfy customer concerns are selected—the acceptance phase of the exchange cycle (Figure 14.1). This is also Step 1 of the QFD process as presented here. For some organizations, this is all that is needed.

- Next (Figure 14.2), the team identifies what measures of performance they will use to declare their performance to be complete (Figure 14.1)—Step 2. For some organizations, this is sufficient.

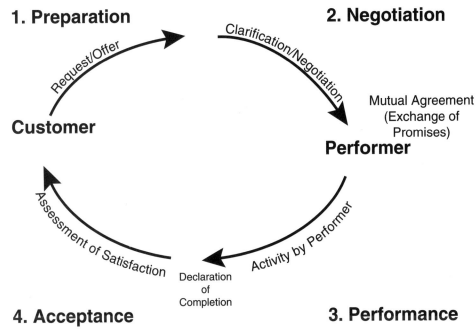

1. Preparation

2. Negotiation

Request/Offer

Clarification/Negotiation

Customer

Mutual Agreement
(Exchange of
Promises)

Performer

Assessment of Satisfaction

Activity by Performer

Declaration
of
Completion

4. Acceptance

3. Performance

Figure 14.1. Action Workflow® The exchange of value. The goal of the project is to create meaning and value for customers.

- Next, the team identifies what actions—key functions—need to be performed—Step 3.

- How might we fail to deliver these demanded qualities, measures, or functions? This is Step 4.

- What internal organizational processes—networks of commitment—are we going to use to deliver these functions? Step 5.

- Who will do what, when, where, and so on? Step 6.

Steps 3 through 6 complete what actions need to be performed by the organization to deliver the conditions of satisfaction—completion of the Performance Phase (Figure 14.1). The organization then can make offers (promises) to customers to fulfill the concern or need:

- How are we going to know we have succeeded from the customer's perspective? This closes the loop.

The QFD process starts by identifying the customer, their needs, and their concerns. This first step cannot be compromised. In Blitz QFD, however, once the three or four most important demanded qualities are identified, the three or four most important performance measures can be estimated as the performance measures most strongly related to the selected demanded qualities. These performance measures are used to evaluate the system being designed. The three or four functions most necessary to perform the selected demanded qualities should then be used for creating the system. Prevention of the failure modes most damaging to the selected demanded

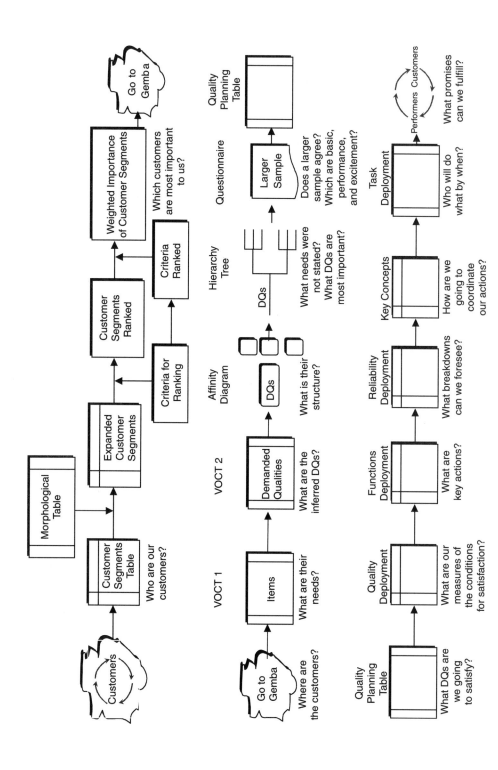

Figure 14.2. A summary flow chart of comprehensive QFD process.

qualities should be included in the system. The tasks necessary for the functions must be included in the systems procedures.

The Office of Technology Assessment (Institute of Medicine 1985) suggests that approximately 80 percent of what is done in the practice of medicine is done out of habit, not science. They define *science* as practices that have data. The minimal threshold for data in their study was experience supported by numbers, for example, a table in a textbook, not randomized controlled clinical trials. Yet even with this minimal definition, only 20 percent of the medical practice was considered evidence-based. There is enormous room for improvement.

Our own experience indicates that quality assurance systems in hospitals are similar. Much of what is done in the name of quality assurance is done out of habit. As isolated problems are identified or a survey occurs and deficiencies are found, corrective action plans and measures to track results are implemented.

More often than not, quality processes have been modified piece by piece to put out fires, not as a design for the whole.

In such a setting, major improvements in quality can occur with relatively simple, well-designed systems. In this case, *well-designed* means "like in the body" starting with the image of an integrated whole. Complexity is then enfolded into the whole as it is needed. We see the possibility of making major improvements in health-care quality using relatively focused efforts that apply the principles of Comprensive QFD and Blitz QFD.

Chapter 15

Epilogue

Upon completion of this chapter, you will have:

- Assessed whether we fulfilled our commitment

- Revisited the issue that the map is not the territory

- Seen why successful change comes from experiencing the environment

In his book *Teaching the Elephant to Dance,* Jim Belasco (1990) describes how trainers shackle young elephants with heavy chains attached to deeply embedded stakes. The elephants pull and tug at the chains but remain attached, and fixed. They learn that they cannot move away. "An older elephant never tries to move farther, even though it has enough strength to pull up the stakes. Its conditioning limits its movement even though it has only a small metal bracelet around its foot, sometimes attached to nothing."

We, like the elephant, view the world based on our earlier conditioning. We are shackled to our historical interpretations. For the most part, we do not question whether the barriers we see are truly limitations imposed by the world or limitations we project onto the world. As infants and children, we experience recurrent patterns in the material world by virtue of our physical interactions within it. We organize our world on the structure of these learned patterns before we learn language. We become aware of our bodies as three-dimensional containers into which we put things (food, water, and air) and out of which things emerge (air, blood, and urine). We also experience physical containment by our surroundings. Through our movements we distinguish space through which movement occurs and time as a measure of movement in space. We move in and out of rooms, clothing, vehicles, and other bounded space. We manipulate objects by placing them into containers and taking them out.

As we acquire language, we learn to translate these patterns of the physical world into symbolic codes: single words, short phrases, and complex narratives (Johnson 1993). In doing so, we unwittingly translate the finiteness and rigidity of our physical world into our social and spiritual dimensions.

$$A \longrightarrow B$$

We talk about the progress of a project from beginning to end as though the project involved moving an object from Point *A* to Point *B* through a space and over time. The end becomes the goal. Impediments to motion along the path become difficulties. We talk about how quickly or slowly the project is going and whether the end is in sight. We talk about close or distant, open or closed, heavy or light, problems that weigh on us, and problems that slow us down.

To illustrate this point, listen to someone describe the significance of an event to another person, especially one who did not witness the event. We use spatial and temporal similes or metaphors to ascribe order and significance. We integrate the myriad of stimuli that are constantly presented to us upon these schema.

THE NATURE OF OUR MAPS OF THE WORLD

Like cells and bodies, our maps of the territory of our social spaces are complex, interconnected wholes. They have structure, internal relationships, patterns for generating and exchanging value, external relationships, and patterns of change. Our mapped social spaces are parts of a system through which we interact with one another, creating new social organizations, communities, and cultures.

The exchange of value and feedback (rewards and consequences) triggers minute-to-minute adaptations within our social networks, creating social homeostasis. When stimulation from the environment overwhelms us, we look to past experience for an effective action. Like in the cell, this process keeps us tied to a past-based future. When we face a situation not experienced in the past, we must shift to being future-based (adapt) or we will suffer.

Adaptation usually requires the development and differentiation of new concepts, new practices, and new habits (learning). Healthy adaptation and differentiation unfold within and in such a way that we remain an integrated and aligned whole.

Like all living systems, be they an amoeba or flatworms in the pond or human beings in an organization, we respond to stimuli from the environment in such a way that we seek what is nurturing and avoid what is noxious. The flatworm over a period of both evolutionary time and individual life span develops instinctual and learned maps (schema) of what is nurturing and noxious. So do we.

We, however, have developed much more specialized sense organs and central processing mechanisms to enact richer maps of our world. Yet, we have come to perceive the map as the territory and not just a map of the world. When we do this, our maps unnecessarily constrain us, and they create confusion. When we focus on the drama on our narrative channel that is frequently triggered by the feedback informing us of the gaps between what we expect and what is showing up, we suffer. We have forgotten that our conceptual maps of the world are built on assumptions or strategies that seemed to work in the past. In forgetting this, we come to believe the assumptions that underlie our worldviews as facts about a world that exists independent of our perception of it. This false belief in the map is fundamental, a root cause, for many of the breakdowns in the social worlds we create together as human beings. This false belief is also a root cause of much of the illness and disease that healthcare providers seek to treat and alleviate. At least seven of the ten most common causes of illness in the United States are preventable by altering lifestyles—lifestyles that often make no sense outside that individual's map.

A SUMMARY OF THE TEXT AS A PROCESS

The promise made to you, the reader, at the beginning of the text was that, if you engaged in the exercises and practices presented, your capacity to diagnose and treat organizational inefficiencies would be greatly enhanced. We have presented a simple picture of the cell and a simple test—the reach test—that makes explicit the essential components necessary for any living, dynamic system. We also briefly listed three challenges that face all organizations, from cells to businesses. They are:

1. Agreeing upon and exchanging value within the environment

2. Managing internal specialization (differentiation) while maintaining organizational alignment (integration)

3. Adapting to rapidly changing environments

We briefly touched on the social issue of world hunger to illustrate how the failures to meet these challenges show up as breakdowns in our organizations. These breakdowns include:

1. Difficulty defining and agreeing upon what is important

2. Our tendency to focus on the immediate, the parts, at the expense of the whole

3. The absence of reinforcing and balancing feedback to nurture efforts of change

These constitutive breakdowns are root causes for many barriers to the delivery of excellence in services. We presented a basic map or cycle that makes explicit the necessary steps to successfully coordinate our actions and exchange value with others. This cycle symbolizes a series of actions and points to phenomena that bind us together within our social units.

Finally, we presented a set of tools and practices—comprehensive QFD—to identify what is important or missing, to set new targets, and to identify measures that are needed to design spaces and processes for successfully meeting challenges and overcoming breakdowns. The initial tools capture and rank data. The data may open up opportunities or challenge our existing organizational beliefs or both. The later tools generate organizational alignment around measures for what is important.

QFD is a series of steps, a process, and an algorithm. It embodies tools that keep what the customer identifies as important (targets) linked to what is actually done within the organization (functions and tasks). When done well, the failure mode deployment and new concept deployment steps build in feedback measures that bring the future to the present for each critical task and integrate the differentiated parts into one whole. The process of QFD can be summarized as follows:

Step 0. What is important to us?[1]
- Identify a service need or concern.
- Identify organizational goals for the project.

Step 1. Customer Deployment—Identifying the Demanded Qualities. What is important?

---

[1]Organization priorities and goals can be sorted and ranked using the same QFD tools used to rank customer needs.

• Identify customers and customer segments.
• Identify criteria to rank segments.
• Identify important customer segments.
• Go to the Gemba.
• Identify important qualities demanded by these customer segments.

Step 2. Quality Deployment—Measuring what is important.
  • Translate the voice of the customer into the voice of the design or redesign team.

Step 3. Function Deployment—Generating what is important.
  • Identify key functions.

Step 4. Failure Mode Deployment. How can/do those functions fail?
  • Identify important failure modes.

Step 5. Concept Deployment—Integrating the parts and organizing the whole, a delivery system.
  • Identify new or more robust processes for delivering the service.

Step 6. Task Deployment—Defining accountability.
  • Who will do what, by when, where, how, and so on?

These steps:

1. Identify what is important
   • Voice of the customer
   • Performance measures for what is important
   • Functions to provide what is important

2. Integrate the parts into a whole
   • A process, a system
   • Failure modes for the process

3. Generate the reinforcing and balancing feedback needed for change
   • Performance measures to assess actions
   • Feedback to critical tasks

We noted that some organizations elect not to use all the steps of QFD but at some point along the journey return to their *as is* processes. We stated that when this is done, it should be done by design—when the process has reached Point 3 on the change map (Figure 2.9)—not by default. We suggest that such a strategy will work consistently only when the *as is* process already embodies mechanisms for direct and formal feedback both from internal and external customers, that is, the environment. This feedback must include performance measures that correlate with the changes in demanded qualities that are targeted by the project to be delivered. Why? Because organizations, like individuals, are systems already functioning in some homeostatic balance. Unless the organization gets feedback that reinforces the desired change, it will use its existing (old) feedback and the rewards and consequences coupled to that feedback, which will reinforce old behavior. Like the staff in the skilled nursing facility distributing "unauthorized" sedative hypnotics, though informed of new goals and the rationale behind them, the organization remained trapped in its old ways.

In chapter 2 we presented a few visual paradoxes and described a few experiments in an attempt to focus your attention on how we have become, trapped in the map versus the territory. We will present some additional data to further substantiate this claim.

THE NATURE OF OUR AWARENESS

The following experiments were carried out in a series of conscious, unanesthetized patients who had previously had electrodes implanted in their brains for treatment of Parkinson's disease or intractable pain. The sensory experiments provide physiological data related to a phenomenon many of you probably experienced as a child when you stared at a colored figure on a page for a few minutes and then looked at a blank, white wall. Behold, after staring at the figure for a few minutes and then looking at the wall, you could still see the figure, an illusionary afterimage. The following experiments support the interpretation that not just this trick but all our phenomenal awareness, both what we call objective and subjective, is an image of what has just occurred, of the past. Our phenomenal awareness is a map we enact through our actions so that, like the amoeba and the flatworm, we can navigate within our ponds. To confuse the map with the territory is to confuse the menu with the meal.

The two categories of experiments that will be presented were carried out by Benjamin Lipet and colleagues (Lipet 1993). The first is a set of three experiments involving perception. The second is a set that involves our motor actions and our sense of a self as the initiator of our actions. The experiments inquire into the nature of our awareness of our worlds and our awareness of phenomena. Our phenomenal awareness is generated through our primary senses (sights, sounds, etc.) and our internal bodily sensations. It is shaped by our conceptual understanding of the external world, linguistic distinctions, and internally generated images. *Phenomenal awareness* as used here is distinct from what is usually called *intuition*. The experiments inquire into the processes by which we generate our maps of the world of phenomena. Why the concern with maps? Our actions in the world are affected by the maps we embody. Ineffective maps yield ineffective actions. Overly rigid maps constrain change.

To carry out the following experiments, Lipet could not simply ask the person when they were aware, because this would involve time for processing the question and initiating a second action. Instead, Lipet took advantage of a special clock. This clock was on an oscilloscope. A red dot rotated around the oscilloscope in a 360-degree pattern, but did so in 2.56 seconds instead of the 60 seconds of our usual clock. The arc that would correspond to 10 seconds on a normal clock equaled 0.2 second on the oscilloscope. Subjects watched the clock, and, when they experienced a sensation or noted they were about to move, they noted the position of the dot and reported its position at the time of this awareness.

If an area of the body, say a portion of the hand, was stimulated with a series of electrical shocks, the subject reported feeling the sensations about 20 milliseconds after the onset of the shock. Electrodes placed over the scalp or directly on the area of the brain corresponding to the hand recorded a response (Figure 15.1). The onset of the first major negative peak was about 20 milliseconds, the entire response about 500 milliseconds.

The sensations that arise in the body, including the hand, are carried by the sensory pathways (Figure 15.2). The pattern is similar to that which we saw for vision (see Figure 2.2) . There is a receptor in the periphery of the body. An axon travels to the brainstem and there connects to its second border neuron, which goes to an area of the brain called the thalamus. From the thalamus, the pathway travels to the cerebral cortex, the area where we believe the sensation is processed.

In patients with chronic pain, electrodes are sometimes implanted in the thalamus as a way of treating pain. Electrodes can also be placed on the surface of the cortex. In

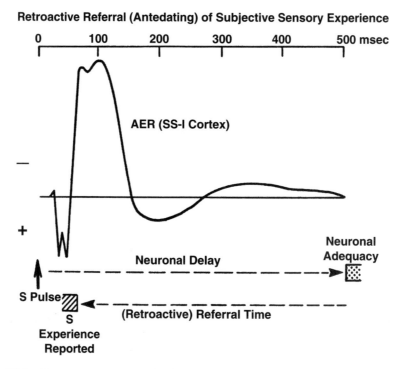

Figure 15.1. Somatosensory evoked potentials. The average evoked response (AER) recorded over the sensory cortex was obtained by applying single pulses just above threshold to a portion of the contralateral hand. This results in a somatosensory evoked potential. The onset of activity occurs at approximately 20 milliseconds, and the entire response takes about 500 milliseconds.

Source: B. Lipet et al., "Subjective Referral of the Timing for a Conscious Sensory Experience: A Functional Role for the Somatosensory Specific Projection System in Man," *Brain* 102 (1979): 199–201. Oxford, U.K.: Oxford University Press. Used with permission.

a series of experiments where the surface of the cortex was stimulated directly through such electrodes, 500 milliseconds of stimulation was required before awareness occurred (Figure 15.3).

So how is it that it takes 500 milliseconds of activity in the brain to appreciate the sensation, yet we can experimentally show that the sensation is experienced within 20 milliseconds when the hand is stimulated? Lipet postulated that our experience of the sensation is projected "back in time"; our awareness of the sensation is projected back so that it seems to have occurred 20 milliseconds after the onset of the peripheral stimulus, even though it will take another 480 milliseconds of brain activity for us to become consciously aware of the stimulus. In some ways, this is not dissimilar to the results from staring at a figure and then looking at the wall. These experiments suggest that awareness of a phenomenon, like the afterimage, occurs after the fact and that our maps of time are something we create or enact.

A second set of perceptual experiments supported this hypothesis. In these experiments, a subliminal stimulus was applied to the skin and then a central stimulus was subsequently applied either in the thalamus or on the sensory cortex. A *subliminal stimulus*

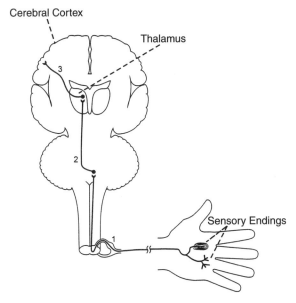

Figure 15.2. Pathways for somatosensory evoked potentials. Like the visual system, receptors are stimulated in the skin. Impulses carrying information are transmitted centrally to the ventral lateral nucleus (VLN) of the thalamus. From here the final neuron projects to the sensory portion of the surface of the brain, the cortex. In the experiments described in the text, the stimulation of either the ventral lateral nucleus of the thalamus or the surface cortex required 500 milliseconds of activity to produce a response that the subject became aware of in their phenomenal awareness.

Source: B. Lipet et al., "Subjective Referral of the Timing for a Conscious Sensory Experience: A Functional Role for the Somatosensory Specific Projection System in Man," *Brain* 102 (1979): 199–201. Oxford, U.K.: Oxford University Press. Used with permission.

is one below the threshold at which we ordinarily detect any sensation. Interestingly, when the central stimulation was applied alone, the subject would not become aware of the sensation until 500 milliseconds of activity, but when the central stimulation was paired with subliminal, peripheral stimulation, the subject's awareness occurred at 20 milliseconds, supporting Lipet's hypothesis.

In another series of experiments, subjects were given subliminal stimuli on the skin, such as the back of the hand. The subjects were then asked to respond to two questions. First, they were forced to answer *yes* or *no* to whether they thought they had received the stimulus; second, they were asked whether they were aware, not aware, or uncertain whether they received the stimulus or not. Up to 75 to 80 percent of the time when the subjects were not "consciously" aware of the phenomenon of being stimulated, they were able to correctly guess whether they had or had not received a stimulus.

These experiments suggest that much of our awareness of the world and our subsequent actions can be carried out without ever reaching our phenomenal awareness. This should not be surprising. You have probably had the experience of unexpectedly touching something hot, such as a hot stove, and already having pulled your finger back before you were aware of the sensation of hotness or burning. Another example would be when something flies toward your face and you begin to close your eyes and duck, but it is only after these actions have been initiated that are you aware of what the flying object was.

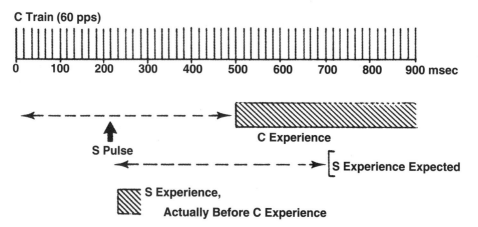

Figure 15.3. Subjective time of cerebrally induced versus skin-induced sensations. As shown in the figure, when the skin is stimulated, the person's awareness of the sensation appears to them to occur at a time approximately 20 milliseconds after the stimulus. In contrast, when the stimulus is applied centrally either in the VLN of the thalamus or the surface of the cortex, the awareness does not appear until 500 milliseconds after the stimulus. In another series of experiments (not shown), when a subliminal stimulus is applied to the skin, of which the person would normally have no phenomenal awareness, and then a central stimulus is applied, the person experiences the central stimulus as arising at a time approximately 20 milliseconds after the subliminal (peripheral) stimulus was applied.

Source: B. Lipet et al., "Subjective Referral of the Timing for a Conscious Sensory Experience: A Functional Role for the Somatosensory Specific Projection System in Man," *Brain* 102 (1979): 199–201. Oxford, U.K.: Oxford University Press. Used with permission.

Motor tasks such as driving the car and walking are other examples. We do not consciously become aware of all the actions necessary to carry out these tasks.

In "blind-sight" experiments, subjects who have lost a portion of their vision because of injury to the visual cortex of the brain indicate they are able to correctly identify shapes and colors in the areas in which they cannot "consciously" see. These findings are consistent with those of the preceding experiments. The awareness of the perceptions as a visual image or map was lost but the prephenomenal awareness was not. These studies are consistent with the notion that our phenomenal maps are at least in part feedback about what has just occurred.

The second category of experiments carried out by Lipet and colleagues had to do with motor activity. Before we initiate an action, such as movement of the finger, electrical activity can be recorded over the surface of the brain. This is called the *readiness action potential,* and it begins approximately 500 milliseconds before the onset of spontaneous motor action. Lipet designed a series of experiments to identify when we are actually aware that we are going to move within the 500-millisecond readiness action potential (Figure 15.4).

Subjects were asked to initiate a motor activity, such as moving their index finger, and to note when they were aware that they were going to move using the position of the red dot on the clock described earlier. Just as in earlier experiments, the position on

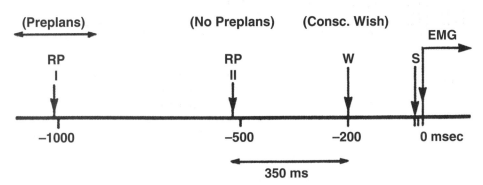

Figure 15.4. Sequence of events and awareness of a fully self-initiated voluntary act. The horizontal axis is time. Time *0* is the time muscle activity (measured by EMG) is detected. The *RP* (rediness potential) begins at approximately 1000 milliseconds when some preplanning is reported (*RP I*) or at about 550 milliseconds with spontaneous action lacking immediate preplanning (*RP II*). Subjective impairment of the wish to move (*W*) appears at about −200 milliseconds, some 300 milliseconds after the onset of even an *RP II*, but well before the EMG activity.

Source: B. Lipet, "Neural Time Factor in Perceptions and Free Will," *Revue de Metaphysique et de Morale* 97 (1992): 252. Paris, France: *Revue de Metaphysique et de Morale.* Used with permission.

the clock was used to measure time. In these motor experiments, people were not aware that they were about to move until 300 milliseconds into the readiness action potential or until 200 milliseconds before the actual movement. That is, the brain was already engaged in electric activity to move the finger before the subjects were even aware they were about to move. What does this say about our common sense notion about initiating our actions? Clearly, when we become aware of our actions to move, we are already in the process of acting and we have 200 milliseconds before the action occurs to continue with that action or to abort it. Our awareness is an awareness of actions we are already doing; it is feedback.

Taken together, this series of sensory and motor experiments indicates that our phenomenal awareness and thoughts are maps of what has just happened. In other words, all thought is a past event. Many of our actions already begin to actively flow prereflectively, before our phenomenal awareness even occurs. The more our actions flow from this level, the more we are aligned with our biology and in harmony with our environment. Our phenomenal awareness is feedback. It is a *product* of our action, not the *initiator* (Figure 15.5). Experimental data from cells and from the human being suggest two-thirds (Figure 15.4) to 95+ percent (Figure 3.6) of activity important to our actions may have already occurred before we are aware we are even going to act.

Our phenomenal map is a complex map, a mixture of perceptions, concepts, moods, and emotions. In one moment, it is a map of what has just happened (feedback); in another moment, it is a map of expectations (targets). Whether perceived as feedback or targets, it is a map like that of Ptolomy's universe, a worldview where we perceive ourselves at the center.

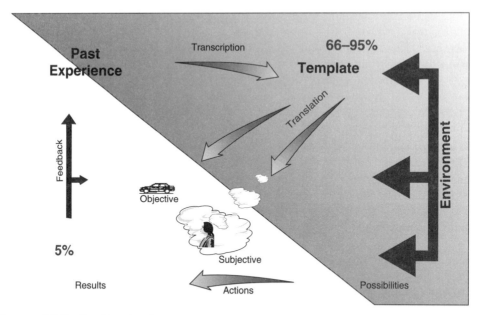

Figure 15.5. Dualism in phenomenal awareness (feedback). Our awareness of the world appears as dividied into subjects and objects. This dualistic awareness is a product of preawareness, prereflective processing. If we were similar to the cell, approximately 95 percent of the activity of our awareness and from where we coordinate our activities would occur before phenomenal awareness of the activity appears. Yet, in our ordinary everyday way of living, we spend 95 percent of our attention focused on actions and the result (feedback) of actions (the moods and emotions) that are a result. Motor experiments would suggest that at least two-thirds of our activity that precedes an action is activity we are not aware of.

When we struggle with the map and with trying to change its contents, we are forgetful that the perceptual and emotive component of the map is built upon assumptions—we are trapped in our self-assumed universe and we suffer. When we live from our constructs of the world, we second-guess or block our direct and innate capacity of knowing—what we commonly call intuition—with our conceptual frameworks built on the past.

The scientific method is not peculiar to science, nor is the PDCA cycle peculiar to quality. Both reflect part of the living process itself. Both by their nature gather data to support or reject assumptions. Yet, in our everyday ordinary perceptual world, we often confine our struggles to the results of our actions and what we judge as their implications and forget to challenge the assumptions that underlie them. We, like the cells in our bodies, are predisposed to past-based futures. We can, however, challenge our embodied assumptions and transcend our tendency to past-based futures by interaction with our environment. The initial portions of the QFD process do just that.

They are designed to focus our attention on stimuli—data—from the environment. Data captured from the environment is ranked in a hierarchy of importance by customers in the environment. The ranking of data and the calculation of the relationship matrices are tools to keep our attention on what is important as we make and challenge our current assumptions and make new assumptions about our actions. Closing the loop with the customer, that is, gathering data that results from deploying our new products and services, after deployment allows us to confirm, reject, or modify our assumptions.

Are you finding these claims outrageous? Recall the split-brain experiments from chapter 3. You already have detailed narratives to explain the world. These narrative maps include a description of the way we operate within the phenomenal world, but this description is itself a product of action and is not the initiator. As noted earlier, we tell and listen to our stories as though they are facts. Once we have a story, we usually do not reexamine the evidence for it, let alone the assumptions it is based on. We tend to interpret new data in terms of what we already know. We tend to fit the data to our story rather than fully attend to what we directly perceive and the potential implications for our worldviews—a worldview that has us at its center. This notion does violence to some of the basic assumptions upon which our common-sense view of the world is built. So did Copernicus's claim that the earth was not the center of the universe.

We are not claiming that what we have presented is fact, the way it really is in the world. We are only presenting an alternative model for looking at the world, one we assess is more effective. However, do not accept our claim, even though it is more consistent with 2500+ years of experience from the perennial wisdom traditions than the traditional Western common sense of today. Be skeptical. Engage in the book and its exercises, engage in a comprehensive QFD project, gather your own data, and then accept or reject our claims. If you do, you too will begin to get feedback from people like "it was the best design project they have ever worked in" (from Appendix F).

In biology, we have amassed a good deal of information about the processes and feedback mechanisms that occur in the cytoplasm of the cell to coordinate the cell's activities. We also have a good deal of data about how the cell captures information from the environment, amplifies this information, and disseminates it throughout the cell. We soon will have maps of the particular sets of actions that each gene encodes. However, we are still relatively naïve in our concepts about how the genetic composition (cell "leadership") selects between the many potential cooperative and competing actions for deployment within the organization. How does the cell decide which stimuli are important enough to initiate change? We are even more in the dark about the coordination of complex relationships between the cells of the body. How do cells and bodies integrate both competition and cooperation while generating overall value for both the parts and the whole?

We face these same conceptual and experiential challenges as our social organizations, communities, and societies unfold. In QFD, we see a set of tools that begin to look at these questions. The Voice-of-the-Customer Table, customer surveys, and the Analytical Hierarchy Process are practices to capture data from the environment and identify what is important. The Quality Planning Table is used to set targets. The Demanded Qualities/Performance Measures Matrix translates these targets into organizational performance measures, which are used to identify key functions, critical paths, and important feedback to both integrate what is important throughout the entire process into the present and to provide feedback by which to navigate. These tools are catalysts that facilitate progress on the archetypal journey of change. These are the strategies that can be used to reduce the energy required to shift an organization from Point 2 to Point 3 (Figure 2.9).

If the service being evaluated is already assessed as functioning well, the goal is to obtain data from the customers. Translating this customer information into performance measures, monitoring the results, and initiating self-correcting mechanisms may be all that is needed. If, on the other hand, the process must include a major shift in perspective or cultural change, as in many of the problems that currently face healthcare, it is important to identify new functions, new critical tasks, potential failure points, and feedback that will build the space in which change can emerge.

A common question is, "How much time should be devoted to a QFD project?" The response is, "That depends." It depends upon the complexity of the project, the number of people involved, and the competitiveness of the environment. It depends upon the complexity and the number of maps you are trying to change. It depends on whether the project is aligned with the ongoing inertia of the organization or service or sets a new direction.

The principles embodied in QFD can be applied during relatively brief encounters. When a patient comes in to see a physician, the experienced and efficient physician goes through something akin to the QFD process. He or she identifies the concerns of the patient, obtains information about symptoms and signs in order to identify a breakdown or breakdowns in the patient's body or social environment, and then identifies overall strategies or functions that will be deployed by carrying out specific tasks. These strategies include observable or measurable feedback measures.

The case study took three and a half months. Building a new automobile may take three years. In any event, the principles embodied in QFD are strategies you already use every moment of every day from the cells in your body to the work you do through social encounters. The goal of this text has been to make the practice explicit so that you can see, feel, and use it more successfully.

Unlike cells in the human body, where the genetic map can only change generation to generation and innovation is usually cancerous, we can change the maps of our social bodies within our lifetime. We do this primarily through perturbations from the environment. As for the cell in our bodies, most of the perturbations to our social organizations are blunted by biological and sociohomeostatic mechanisms. When these mechanisms are overwhelmed or prove inadequate, we search for appropriate memory files of our past successes while trying to avoid our past failures. Only when we have exhausted all of these are we truly open to change. Occasionally we encounter paradoxes or anomalies in our maps. When these are shaped by the environment to address some environmental concern and are subsequently adopted as a practice, we call them innovations. We present QFD as one possible way to capture stimuli from the environment and incorporate these perturbations to either change our current maps or to shape anomalies into innovations and produce meaning and value. The strategies and practices presented here are a series of actions catalyzed by tools to shift the organizational attention and behavior from self-centered maps to customer-oriented maps, be the customer on individual, another organization or a community, or an ecosystem. The tools are about putting service above self and providing value for the community.

Appendix A

Sample Forms

These samples can be copied and used as worksheets.

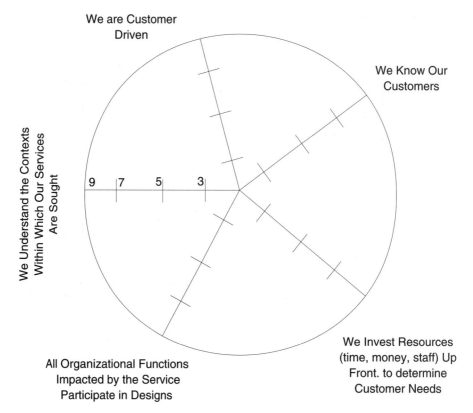

Figure A.1.

Project Schedule

Start Date								
Phase	Purpose	Tasks	Who	When	How	Document

Phase	Purpose	Tasks	Who	When	How	Document
Check Current Market		C: A: P: D:				
Act		C: A: P: D:				
Plan		C: A: P: D:				
Do		C: A: P: D::				
Check		C: A: P: D::				

Figure A.2.

Voice of Customer Table I

Customer Info	Voice of the Customer I	Who, What, When, Where	Why	How	Reworded Data
		Who What When Where			
		Who What When Where			
		Who What When Where			
		Who What When Where			
		Who What When Where			

Figure A.3.

Voice of the Customer Table 2

Customer ID	Demanded Quality	Performance Measure	Function	Reliability	Failure Modes	Other Failures

Figure A.4.

235

Quality Planning Table

Demanded Qualities	Important—AHP Field	Customer Importance Rating	Customer Competitive Evaluations				Targets and Weighted Demanded Qualities Composite				Composite Importance as %
			Our Organization	Competitor 1	Competitor 2	Competitor 3	Target	Ratio of Improvement	Sales Points	DQ Composite Importance	
1.											
2.											
3.											
4.											
5.											
6.											
7.											

Figure A.5.

House of Quality

Performance Measures

Demanded Qualities	Customer Importance Rating									Our Oganization	Competitor 1	Competitor 2	Competitor 3	Target	Ratio of Improvement	Sales Points	DQ Composite Improtance
1.																	
2.																	
3.																	
4.																	
5.																	
6.																	
7.																	
Weighted Priorities																	
Desired Targets																	

Figure A.6.

Performance Measures/Functions Matrix

Functions

	Units of Measure							
	Target							
	Performance Measure Weight							

Performance Measures

Weight Concepts

Figure A.7.

238

Functions/Failure Modes Matrix

Functions Modes

Functions

Weighted									

Figure A.8.

New Concepts Matrix

AHP Weighting				
Constraints				

Figure A.9.

240

Task Deployment Table

What	Who	When	Where	How	How Much	Why	Other

Figure A.10.

Appendix B
Glossary of Phrases

This is an example of what a Glossary might look like.

Demanded Qualities	Customer Statements
More comprehensive evaluations	Diagnostic medical evaluations are comprehensive and complete (no surprises later).
More comprehensive reports	Reports are both comprehensive and complete (i.e., "no loose ends").
Definition of all findings as pre- or postinjury	Preexisting factors of impairment and disability are clearly separated from those of injury.
Better work capacity assessments	Assessments of current work capacities and limitations are more detailed.
More MD follow-through with recommendations	Recommendations are implemented by workers' treating physicians.
More acceptance of findings at hearings	Reports withstand challenge during administrative hearings.
Independence from insurers maintained	You are perceived as independent from the insurer.
More understandable reports	Findings and conclusions are able to be understood by a layperson.

Performance Measures	Teams Definition
% Symptoms identified	Final report to list symptoms (numerator) and requests for etiology and so on of symptoms on follow-up denominator. A symptom is every statement expressing a change in capability, feeling, confidence, and so on made by a patient.
% Findings identified	Final report to list abnormal findings (numerator) and requests for etiology and so on of findings on follow-up denominator. An abnormal finding is any deviation from normal of a physical characteristic, laboratory, or radiological study.
% Treatments identified	Final report to list treatments (denominator) and requests for etiology and so on of treatments on follow-up numerator. A treatment is any intervention to change a finding or a symptom including perception items, medical procedures, over-the-counter medications, or alternative medicine practices.

% Findings linked to observable data	Count of findings and observable data to support findings, observable data, evidence, is any observation of function or behavior that could be witnessed by an appropriately trained profession, or laboratory, radiological or operative data.
% Findings separated into industrial or nonindustrial	Counts of all findings and of findings opined as industrial versus nonindustrial over all findings. Industrial is any symptom or impairment that occurs following the injury and can be ascribed to have arisen as a result of the injury. Nonindustrial requires the symptom or impairment to have been present prior to the injury or if it appears after the injury has clearly arisen for factors unrelated to the injury.
% Job requirements simulated and tested	Count of job requirements and number actually simulated and tested. Requirements are those functions or activities that are included in the person's job description or if self-reported by the patient have been verified as part of duties by the employer.
% Capacities and impairments quantified or semi-quantified	Count of impairments graded on scale over count of total impairments. An impairment is any loss of function or a restriction of function as a result of a symptom or finding.
% Workers' treating MDs included in process	Count of currently treating MDs actually contacted over all currently treating MDs.
% Returned to work	% Returned to work at follow-up sampling.
Number unexplained inconsistencies between observers	Count of unexplained inconsistencies between observers.

Appendix C

Taguchi's Loss Function

Many quality discussions have an underlying assumption that quality is a step function. Outside some acceptable boundaries the customer is equally unhappy, and within the range the customer is equally happy (Figure C.1). The vertical axis graphically plots increased displeasure of the customer. The horizontal axis shows the performance being considered. A medical example might be resting heart rate. Heart rates too low are not desirable. Heart rates too high are also not desired, that is, a step pattern of what is best.

In the 1950s, Dr. Genichi Taguchi noted that, in practice, performance measures and customer satisfaction were not simple step functions; rather, as the performance of a system deviated from some target, the customer became proportionally less satisfied. Instead of a step function, a quadratic curve better represents the customer's satisfaction/dissatisfaction, as shown in Figure C.2.

In the figure, both the traditional step function and the smooth quadratic curve are shown. The farther from the target value (shown on the horizontal axis), the less happy the customer. This curve represents what is called "the target-is-best loss function." As performance deviates from the target, there is a loss of customer satisfaction. It is also possible to attach a financial cost to the loss. Attaching cost to the function can be used to cost-justify one system over another. This is beyond this text and not necessary for comparing systems.

Most parameters or performance measures for a service are "larger-is-better" (Figure C.3) or "smaller-is-better" (Figure C.4) relationships.

For *larger-is-better* relationships, customer satisfaction falls from dissatisfied at low levels of the service measure and satisfaction increases as the measure of performance increases. An example of a larger-is-better performance would be the level of comprehensiveness of the patient's evaluation. The more comprehensive the evaluation, the more satisfied the customer. The relationship is not linear. As performance further increases, the incremental increase in customer satisfaction is less. When cost is added to such a function, the interrelationship between incremental satisfaction, incremental performance, and incremental cost can be evaluated. For some services, taking on the additional cost for improving performance produces only marginal increases in customer satisfaction and is not justified. Resources might be better allocated to another service or system. An example of a *smaller-is-better* performance measure is the time required to complete patient's evaluation.

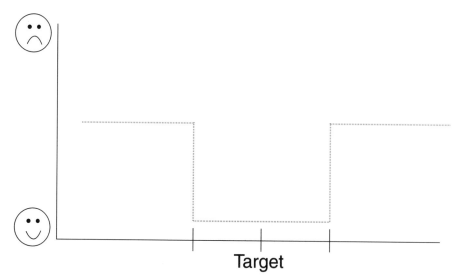

Figure C.1.

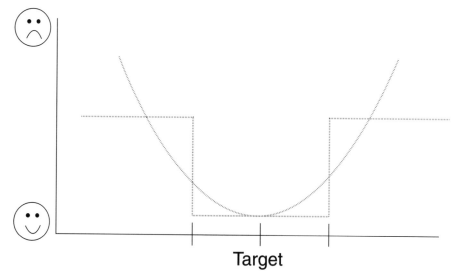

Figure C.2.

TARGET IS BEST AND LOWER VARIATION IS BEST

The implications of Taguchi's findings are that when evaluating competing systems, both the variance and the average performance of the systems must be considered. If the two systems have the same variation but different averages (Figure C.5), the one (A) closest to the target is best. Here the system with the average closest to the target is best.

If two systems have the same averages but different variation, then the one with less variation (A) is preferred (Figure C.6).

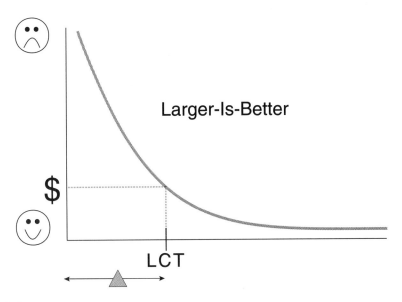

Figure C.3.

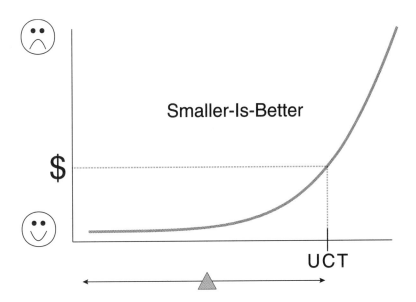

Figure C.4.

If neither the variation nor the average is the same, it is difficult to identify the best system by just looking at the plot (Figure C.7).

In this case, it is necessary to take into account both the deviation of the average from the target for the system and the variation of the system around its average. Here the Mean Square Deviation (MSD) is used as a measure of quality.

$$MS\underline{D} = \sigma^2 + (\bar{y} - T)^2$$

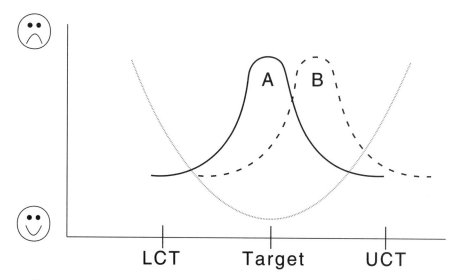

Figure C.5.

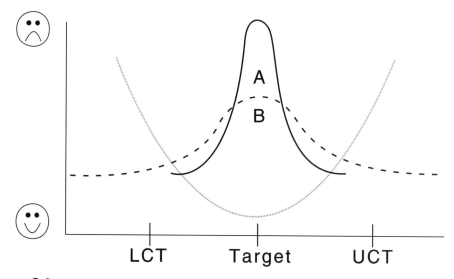

Figure C.6.

The mean square deviation (MSD) is the sum of the variance (standard deviation squared) plus the square of the difference between the target (T) and the average of the system ($\bar{y}$). This calculation incorporates the importance of both variation and average performance for a system. The MSD can be calculated directly by finding the average of the squared deviation from the target.

$$MSD = \frac{\sum\limits_{i=1}^{n}(y_i - T)^2}{n}$$

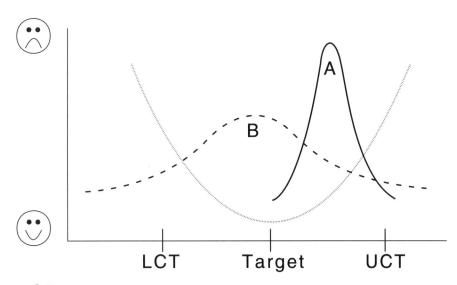

Figure C.7.

n = Number of data recorded
T = Target value
y_i = Individual data points
$y_i - T$ = Deviation of individual data points from the target. These are squared and summed, and the average is found by dividing by n.

When comparing two systems, knowing the variance and the squared deviation is important to understand whether the better system is better because of its variation and/or its average.

As healthcare matures as a service industry and funding moves toward treating the health of groups or communities of people, the principles embodied in Taguchi functions will become more important. For example, consider the Functional Independence Measure (FIM) (Granger et al. 1990), which is a commonly employed performance measure in rehabilitation hospitals. The FIM is an accepted performance measure for the Joint Commission's ORYX initiative. It is used to monitor both individual patient progress and the performance of the organization for a population of patients. Assume a rehab hospital redesigns how services are delivered, for example, for a group of orthopedic patients following joint replacement. Also assume that the mean level of function as measured by the FIM is higher for the six months after implementing a new design versus six months before. Usually, we assume the system with the higher average to be the better. What if we look at the variation and see that the system with the higher average actually has a much wider or a skewed variation. It is possible under the new system, although the average was higher and some people did better, the variation is also much wider and the number of patients with low scores could actually increase. There for the overall customer satisfaction or health of the community might be less under the system with the higher average. These types of comparisons become more important as more and more standard performance measures for delivering healthcare evolve within the industry.

MSD can also be calculated as already described for both the larger-is-better and the smaller-is-better cases.

Larger-Is-Better

The mean square deviation for Larger-Is-Better is

$$MSD_L = \frac{1 + \frac{3\sigma^2}{\bar{y}^2}}{\bar{y}^2} = \frac{\sum\limits_{i=1}^{n} \frac{1}{y_i^2}}{n}$$

Smaller-Is-Better

The mean square deviation for Smaller-Is-Better is

$$MSD_S = \sigma^2 + \bar{y}^2 = \frac{\sum\limits_{i=1}^{n} y_i^2}{n}$$

Appendix D

TRIZ

OVERVIEW

In 1946, while working as a patent investigator, the Russian scientist Genrich Altshuller began to notice a certain order and direction in the world of patents. Some patents were rather ordinary, but others represented a significant change in an existing system. In the latter group of patents, he noted repeating patterns in the solutions to problems that were patented. He also noted that the changes in evolution of the different technical systems over time had some commonalties in their direction. Like the classical biologist, Altshuller identified classes of generic solutions to particular types of problems within technical systems, and he identified directions of evolution for the systems as a whole. Altshuller's insights have developed into a methodology that has become known as the Theory of Inventive Problem Solving (TRIZ). Several analytical tools and knowledge-based tools have evolved during the more than 50 years of development of TRIZ in Russia.

Altshuller identified 40 classes or generic solutions to conflicts with systems, and he identified eight basic patterns that describe the evolution of technical systems (Terninko 1998). These 40 different classes or generic schema of change were found to explain the most innovative types of patents. These have come to be called *the 40 principles.* The eight basic patterns describe the evolution of technical systems and are described as follows.

It is our claim that these basic patterns identified for the evolution of technical systems are not peculiar to machines but rather are expressions of human learning and human conception. In the future, we will come to see that these same patterns underlie the evolution of our systems for services as well. We are presenting a brief introductory overview to the eight patterns of evolutions of systems as these become important in the Functions, Failure Modes, and New Concepts steps in QFD.

EVOLUTION OF TECHNICAL SYSTEMS

1. Stages of evolution of a technological system

2. Evolution toward increased ideality

3. Nonuniform development of system elements

4. Evolution toward increased dynamism and controllability

5. Increased complexity followed by simplification

6. Evolution with matching and mismatching elements

7. Evolution toward microlevels and increased use of fields

8. Evolution toward decreased human involvement

Stages of Evolution of a Technological System—The S Curve

The S curve (Figure D.1) is familiar to many people in health care, as this function describes a number of biological processes. Probably the most familiar is the oxygen saturation curve known to all medical students and physicians. This S pattern is also the classic curve of human learning, product life cycles, and population growth.

As seen in Figure D.1, changes in learning or a system's performance initially starts at a slow and gradual rate followed by a period of rapid change, then the slowing down and leveling off of the rate of change. Finally, such as in the case of product or population life cycles, a decline in performance or number occurs.

In TRIZ, the S curve is used to describe evolution of systems at a macrolevel. There is a separate S curve for every performance measure associated with the system. By renewing the history of the system or a particular performance measure, we can see where the system or performance measure is along this S curve of evolution for its current structure. If the performance of the system is plotted and found to have already leveled off, then this particular level of performance or evolution in the system is very late for its current structure. Breakthroughs in the structural design or the performance of the system are likely to be required before creating more value or growth.

It takes time to design new services and systems. Looking at where a service currently sits along the S curve is an indication of what is needed next to improve the function and the performance of the system. To improve a performance measure in the rapidly rising point of the curve often involves minor change, while innovative change is often required along the flatter portion of the curve and requires substantial change.

To remain competitive, organizations need to develop new options—new designs—before reaching maturity. The S curve then becomes a report card on the system's level of maturity for each of its performance measures.

Evolution toward Increased Ideality

As systems evolve, they become more ideal with respect to their target—their purpose. Every improvement in a system has useful effects and associated cost and harmful effects. The measure of the ideality of a system's design can be considered as the ratio of the useful effects divided by the cost and harmful effects. Harmful effects might include simple things like patient inconvenience, pages of paperwork, or more serious events such as injury or death.

$$\text{Ideality} = \frac{\Gamma \text{ Useful effects}}{\Gamma \text{ Costs } + \Gamma \text{ Harmful effects}}$$

As systems evolve toward ideality, the ratio of useful effects to cost and harmful effects rises. The ideal system provides the desired function without the system; that is, the ideal system performs at least one useful function, but the denominator approaches 0.

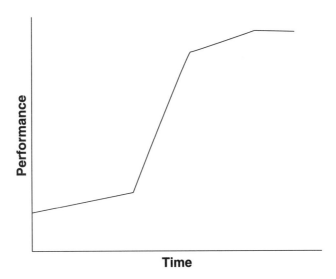

Figure D.1.

For example, a part of health-care delivery in a hospital system includes a departmental supervisor's monitoring of quality of care delivered by the staff to patients. This quality assurance is a useful function. As already noted, one way of moving toward ideality is to improve a function but reduce or remove the part that performs the function. Patients and families could be given copies of treatment plans and educated as to what is expected of them and the staff. This becomes a treatment contract. Patients and families, a resource already within the system, can perform part of the quality assurance function, improving system performance and decreasing the costs and need of managerial supervision to determine if the organization is meeting its commitments.

In an early chapter, we mentioned that one of the main sources of variation in health care today is the variability in performance between physicians for a similar problem and also with a particular physician for a series of similar cases. Currently, large information technology infrastructures are being built and being embraced to make available demographic information, laboratory studies, historical information, and so on. Altshuller's patterns of evolution suggest, once this is in place, that a possible direction for the system as a whole to evolve, with little added cost, will be to eventually have the information infrastructure assume decision-making functions in such a way that will reduce the variation in practice. In every other industry where gross variation has been reduced, quality has improved, cost has been reduced, and harmful effects have been decreased, that is, the system moves toward ideality.

There are several strategies to improving the ideality:

1. Increase the number of desired effects.

2. Increase the performance of the existing desired effects.

3. Do nothing to the desired effects but reduce the cost and harmful effects.

4. Do 1, 2, and 3 all at the same time.

5. Increase the useful effects faster than the cost and harmful effects. This is the classic cost-benefit analysis.

Option 5 should be approached with caution. Attempts to increase the useful effect faster than costs and harmful effects, that is, without addressing factors that contribute to costs, push the system without altering the fundamentals of the system. Unintended consequences, like the lactic acid production in the untrained body that assumes the role of the sprinter, often appear during a later timeframe. For example, Medicare and Medicaid were introduced in the 1960s to improve health care of the population (increase useful effects) without altering the underlying system for delivering care. The true cost of the Medicare/Medicaid system was never fully funded. These unfunded costs were shifted to people with private insurance. This eventually led to the rapid increase in premium rates for private health-care insurance to the extent that many people who had previously had private health insurance could not afford health-care insurance. A large population of uninsured working people emerged, creating another crisis or harmful effect.

The federal government has consistently tried to increase the services (useful effects) to nursing home residents through regulation, that is, it has tried to improve useful effects faster than costs. But these regulations generate unfunded costs that are being shifted to people who pay their way. The cost to be in a nursing home for people who pay themselves is now sometimes 50 percent higher than Medicaid rates.

Nonuniform Development of System Elements

Each subsystem within the larger system has its own rate of maturation or S curve, that is, the time line to maturity of the part is different for each of the subsystems. This results in different subsystems becoming the bottleneck or rate-limiting step in the overall performance of the system at different points during a maturation of the system. A bottleneck or rate-limiting step is that portion of the system or subsystem that prevents the overall system from achieving higher levels of performance. Many organizations continue to allocate resources to a subsystem long after another subsystem or part has become the bottleneck or rate-limiting step. This is often done out of habit or because of psychological inertia.

For example, several years ago a community hospital installed an automated information system. The system was designed such that it could only be used with a touchtone phone. Only 40 percent of the hospital's community had touchtone phones. Lack of touchtone phones in the community was the weak link in the overall system. Improving features in the system itself would not necessarily improve the overall function of the system whose purpose was community access without first increasing the number of touchtone phones in the community.

Evolution toward Increased Dynamism and Controllability

We have all experienced a gatekeeper in a system at sometime or another. The gatekeeper will not allow anything to happen unless a particular sequence of events occurs. A gatekeeper is one strategy for controlling a system. This strategy, however, builds in a certain amount of rigidity, limiting the system's capacity to respond to different settings or changing demands. If we flowcharted such a system, there would be no branches or options at the level of the gatekeeper. An alternative design would be to increase the number of options at the level of the gatekeeper, creating a more dynamic and responsive system. Here, the system and the users automatically select the correct path. The structure of the gatekeeper is removed, and the function is carried out by the dynamism alternatives within the system itself.

Traditional phone companies have a strong gatekeeper history. Traditionally, the phone companies wanted to route calls through particular sets of switches so that they could charge for the bits of data flowing through the switches. The Internet has changed the paradigm. The availability of broad-band, interconnected systems with multiple ways of transmitting information has increased the dynamism of the system, reduced costs, and increased the useful effect. In such systems, people are charged by the amount of time they use the system rather than by the specific amount of data they push through.

Increased Complexity Followed by Simplification

Initially, most systems emerge to provide one function. Over time, often somewhat randomly and haphazardly, additional functions are added. Performance and the appearance of the total system during this march of evolution become increasingly complex and complicated. Redesigning the system toward simplification usually begins with identifying and reducing redundancies and then eliminating them. The higher-level purpose of all systems is used to identify which subsystems/functions/services fit into the new whole.

A particular clinic may start with very specific goals, for example, treating feet. Over time, other services need to be added. They might involve education for diet, stress modification, and then buying shoes. Alternative medicine practices may be introduced, such as rolfing and yoga. This progression eventually can evolve into an organization—a total system—designed to support and facilitate the feet by addressing the entire body. In such a clinic, the boundaries between the formerly separate disciplines and practitioners become increasingly blurred and eventually disappear.

Evolution with Matching and Mismatching Elements

Systems can evolve by adding elements. These elements can be unmatched, matched, or mismatched or have both dynamic matching and mismatching. In our age of symmetry, asymmetrical or mismatching parts or systems are often seen as undesirable. However, asymmetry can enhance features of the system. For example, asymmetrical and irregular spacing of the treads on snow tires markedly reduces the sound vibrations generated by snow tires on pavement.

Consider the example of the evolution of operative procedures for coronary artery disease. Initially, all operative procedures were carried out by surgeons:

1. Unmatched: In the beginning, of course, there were no open heart surgeons. It was only later with time that this evolved as a specialty. Initially teams were put together in a haphazard manner. They included surgeons whose interest in the procedure was more the driving force than their particular discipline.

2. Matched elements: As specially trained cardiac surgeons became more available, the surgical team was composed of all specialists.

3. Mismatched elements: Entirely matched or specialized teams tend to focus and see the problem from a particular perspective. Adding a clinical nurse to such a team expanded the awareness of the team of the patient's needs as a whole as the perspective of nursing, which traditionally looks at the patient as more of a whole, was added to the team.

4. Dynamic matching and mismatching: Now the composition of such teams includes not only various specialists but also various technologies and operative procedures to treat the problem. For example, patients presenting

with acute angina or recurrent angina are first evaluated for angioplasty and cardiac stents, before undergoing coronary bypass surgery, competing or mismatched elements.

Evolution toward Microlevels and Increased Use of Fields

Systems by their nature embody synergies and conflicts. Over time, as a system matures, changes in the system that reduce conflicts focus more and more at the microlevel of the system. Resources (fields) already within the system often become employed and utilized to reduce conflicts at these microlevels.

For example, the rehabilitation process starts by setting broad outlines and goals for a patient. The rehabilitation team consists of multiple disciplines who, following our human tendency to focus on what is immediately before us as described earlier, tend to focus on their particular area of specialty. The continuing challenge in rehabilitation is getting the parts—the disciplines—to focus on the whole—the overall patient, family, and community environment. If we look at ways of enhancing the synergy or reducing these problems within the system at the microlevel, we identify the patient and family as parts of the system and potential resources (fields). Patients and families can be given a detailed treatment plan and become monitors for whether the parts are working toward the larger whole.

Evolution toward Decreased Human Involvement

Social technical systems by their nature evolve to perform repetitive or tedious functions. Over time, as these functions become more rote or automated, less human involvement is required.

Currently, every time a patient enters any point in the health-care system, the same demographic and insurance data is collected in a redundant, complicated fashion. At each point of entry, this is entered into the computer. An enormous amount of human involvement is required for collecting demographic data on patients, collecting insurance data, billing, filing forms for insurance companies, charting routine functions, and so on. As the same information infrastructure has allowed the phenomenal growth of productivity in manufacturing, and the Internet penetrates and moves into health care, much of this activity could be performed at one point in the system and be available to other parts. As the amount of human involvement in this duplication throughout the systems is reduced, it will allow reduction of cost, and ideally, it will increase human resources to address person-to-person the personal contact aspect of providing health care.

Automation of rote procedures, such as reading pap smears, provide another example. Automated systems to read pap smears have already been shown to be more effective and efficient than systems that rely totally on the human and a microscope.

IMPLICATIONS FOR QFD

The traditional approach to creativity is to attempt to jump from "my problem" to "my solution." However, with this strategy there is often no repeatable path from "my problem" to "my solution" and any attempt to follow that route, that is, recreate such past-based futures, could result in a never-ending series of random trials. So, what seems to be a direct approach can take a lifetime.

Through the use of the tools of TRIZ in the design and manufacturing of technical equipment (i.e., mechanical systems), the experiential knowledge generated by past

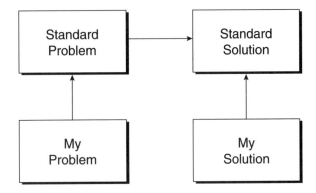

Figure D.2.

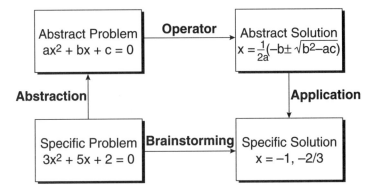

Figure D.3.

solutions has become organized into standard formats or databases. Designers seek to match the problem or conflict they are experiencing to similar conflicts with historical solutions in the database. To do so, the inventor first attempts to translate his particular problem into the language of the standard problem, looks for a standard solution, and then applies the standard solutions to those particular problems (Figure D.2).

For example, consider the problem of solving a specific quadratic equation (Kaplan 1996). The trial and error process is very slow and imprecise; you may never get there. We do not try to brainstorm solutions to quadratic equations. We use a methodology. The specific quadratic equation is translated into generic or standard form. The operation is carried out at the level of the abstract or standard solution, and then the result is translated to your specific problem (Figure D.3).

In the future, health-care organizations and perhaps the industry as a whole will develop databases of standard solutions to particular problems. The Joint Commission on Accreditation of Health-Care Organizations' development of a sentinel event policy is an attempt, much as is done in aviation, to do so. It is a step in that direction. In the meantime, the patterns of evolutions of systems and many of the strategies of TRIZ can already be applied to solving conflicts with our systems of service.

Appendix E

Case Study Complex Evaluation

This appendix presents some details of the case example from chapter 4 and used to illustrate the process of QFD in Part 2 of the text. What is presented here, however, differs somewhat from what has already been presented. The difference comes from three major sources. First, in the text the goal was to present the process of QFD, not the case. The case as presented in the text was simplified and "idealized" to emphasize the theory and steps of QFD. Second, some differences result from practice versus theory. Like models of organizational theory, models of organizational change, or tools for business process design and redesign, QFD is based on a model. Models by their nature are simplified and idealized. Elegant models when fully appreciated flow with a grace and beauty. When applied in practice, however, things often unfold in a very different manner. They are often messy. Results are usually delivered only after a great deal of effort and struggle against organizational, team, and/or individual inertia and other moods and emotions. If this were not the case, the problems more likely than not would have already resolved themselves without any need for special effort or projects. The third source of difference is experience versus the naïveté of the beginner. Just as the infant learns to walk only through stumbling and falling, this was the first QFD case in the organization in which it occurred. The project was carried out without the presence of an outside consultant or facilitator.

We are presenting this case both to illustrate in more detail the process of QFD to the serious student or practitioner and to make it available as a case study to learn from. We will comment on some of the differences between theory and practice and leave the identification of others to the reader.

The team deviated or made "mistakes" relative to the theory and current practice of QFD, yet achieved a seemingly good outcome. This is a comment on both the robustness of QFD as a process and the general lack of performance measures and clinical services based on habit, not design, which predominates healthcare in general. Healthcare via managed care has become an occupied industry. The conquerors by and large came from outside the industry. Like the Spaniards in the 1500s, the conquerors had clearer targets for their objectives, more reproducible and effective measures of performance, and more functional tools for managing organizations and the industry than indigenous

259

people they conquered. These measures are, however, primarily financial. Healthcare will not be able to return to its roots, its core values, until performance measures to measure the delivery of observable aspects of these values and the business processes that deliver them emerge within the industry to provide a counterbalance to financial measures and provider-focused targets, which currently dominate the industry.

BRIEF OVERVIEW

The example is taken from a QFD project at a rehabilitation hospital that provided complex medical and/or legal evaluations for people with complex and catastrophic injuries or illnesses. The services are low in volume, complex, provider intensive, and expensive. Each patient is different and thus requires a somewhat unique and extensive evaluation. A typical evaluation includes physical capacity assessments, radiological tests such as computerized axial tomography (CAT scan), magnetic resonance imaging (MRI), bone scans, and numerous blood chemistries.

Evaluations are conducted by four to eight physicians from different specialties. Two to three therapy-related evaluations are performed. In addition, the process requires the work of 10 to 25 other staff, including people from nursing, technical support, and administrative support. Activities are coordinated among as many as 10 different business organizations. The suppliers of complex radiological testing and physician evaluations are separate business entities. Almost all requests for this service come from workers' compensation insurers. The goal of the QFD project presented in this appendix was to increase the volume of referrals for the service.

A nine-person project team composed of two nurses, two physicians, an occupational therapist, and three representatives from sales and marketing was formed. The project team was charged with improving and, if possible, introducing distinctive and innovative attributes into the rehabilitation organization's evaluation process to increase volume.

IDENTIFYING THE CUSTOMER SEGMENT

Using brainstorming as a strategy, the team generated a list of potential customers and stakeholders (Figure E.1).

The team chose the criterion *Potential for Repeat Referrals* as the criterion by which to judge the importance of various customer segments. The Analytical Hierarchy Process was used to rank the various customer segments (Figure E.2). Insurers were identified as the customer segment with the highest potential to generate repeat referrals.

GOING TO THE GEMBA

A three-person subgroup of the QFD team went to the field and interviewed claims managers, case managers, and legal personnel to gather data about what the customers want. It is preferable for the entire team to be able to visit the customers in the field. In this case, the group of customers that were being interviewed and that would eventually be assembled to carry out rankings were not from the organization's local community. Because of lodging and air expense, only a three-person subgroup conducted the interviews in the field.

Customer wants were captured by interviewing customers; they were captured and sorted using Voice-of-the-Customer Tables 1 and 2; they were grouped using affinity

```
┌─────┬──────────────────────────────────────┐
│     │  Direct Consumers                    │
│     │       Patients                       │
│     │            Over 65                   │
│     │            Under 65                  │
│     │       Families                       │
│     │            Over 65                   │
│     │            Under 65                  │
│     ├──────────────────────────────────────┤
│     │  Payers                              │
│  C  │       Medicare                       │
│  U  │       MediCal                        │
│  S  │       County Services                │
│  T  │       % Charges                      │
│  O  │       Per Diem                       │
│  M  │       Capitated                      │
│  E  │       Workers' Compensation Insurers │
│  R  ├──────────────────────────────────────┤
│  S  │  Referrals Agents                    │
│     │       Case Managers                  │
│     │       Physicians                     │
│     │       Families                       │
│     │       Skilled Nursing Facilities     │
│     ├──────────────────────────────────────┤
│     │  Physicians                          │
│     │       Treating                       │
│     │       Primary                        │
│     │       Others                         │
│     ├──────────────────────────────────────┤
│     │  Employers                           │
│     │       Attorneys                      │
│     │            Plaintiff                 │
│     │            Defense                   │
└─────┴──────────────────────────────────────┘
```

Figure E.1.

grouping; and they were eventually displayed in a tree hierarchy as shown in Figure E.3. The groupings and the demanded qualities were ranked and weighted using the Analytical Hierarchy Process.

RNs, claims managers, legal personnel, and administrators were interviewed either individually or in groups of three to four. During each interview, one person of the three-person interview team took the lead to ask questions, one took notes, and one observed the overall process. The interviews were conducted in the customer's own environment to provide team members with firsthand experience of how their products or services fit into the customer's work and setting. A total of 30 people were interviewed. Most of the QFD literature recommends a minimum of 15 to 20. Larger numbers do not substantially increase the amount of demanded qualities captured.

A 10-person subgroup of the 30 customers who were initially interviewed was assembled, and, using the affinity method, 61 demanded qualities were grouped and then ranked using the Analytical Hierarchy Process. The customers being interviewed had volunteered their time and were not being compensated. The AHP rankings and the building of the tree with the affinity data were carried on concurrently in one half day.

PRR	Insurers	Physicians	Injured Workers	Attorneys	Insurers	Physicians	Injured Workers	Attorneys	Insurers	Physicians	Injured Workers	Attorneys	Row Sums	%
Insurers	1	5	9	3	1	5	9	3	0.610	0.694	0.450	0.577	2.331	58.28
Physicians	1/5	1	5	1	0.2	1	5	1	0.122	0.139	0.250	0.192	0.703	17.58
Injured Workers	1/9	1/5	1	1/5	0.11	0.2	1	0.2	0.067	0.028	0.050	0.038	0.183	4.58
Plaintiff Attorneys	1/3	1	5	1	0.33	1	5	1	0.201	0.139	0.250	0.192	0.782	19.56
					1.64	7.2	20	5.2	1	1	1	1	4.000	100.00

Figure E.2.

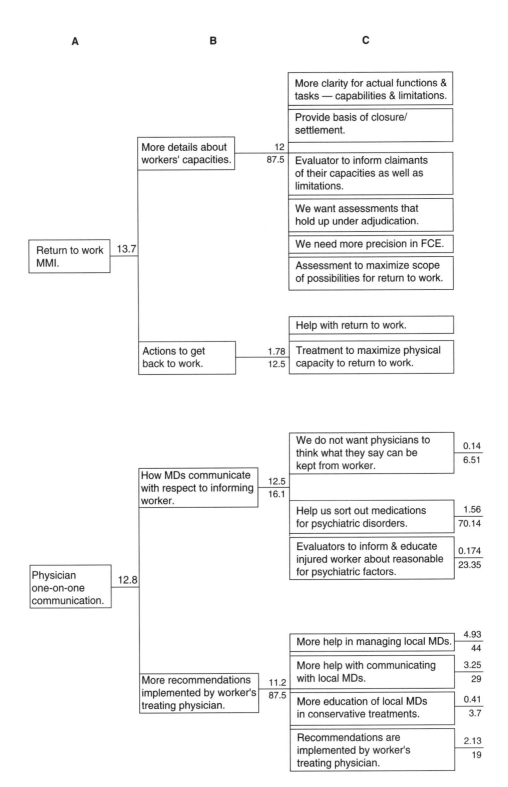

Figure E.3. Part I

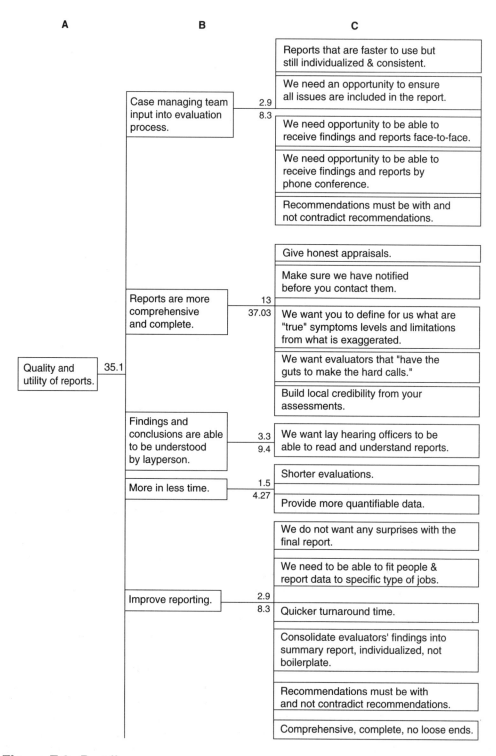

Figure E.3. Part II

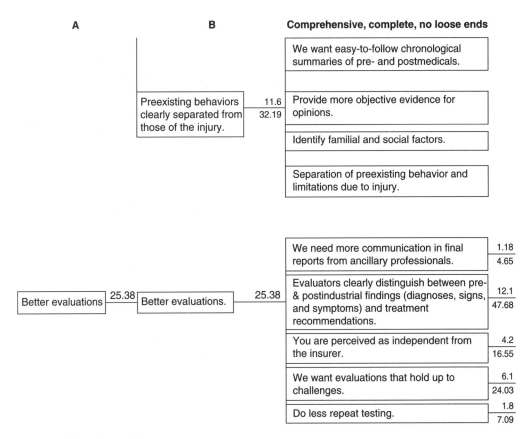

Figure E.3. Part III

During the second round of the affinity grouping, the customers felt that *Better Evaluations,* identified as a label for a group of demanded qualities, was an important enough category that it should not be grouped with another category. When doing the affinity grouping, The team chose Column B from the tree as the level of detail to work with. *Better Evaluations* at Level B did not provide enough detail, however, and the team rationalized that the branches from this level were more probable than not the same level of detail as the other items in Column B. Hence, the team eventually chose three items from this level for the questionnaire.

After returning to their own organization, the team noted some redundancies in the tree. For example, Column B, *Preexisting behaviors clearly separated from those of the injury* and *Evaluators clearly distinguish between pre- and postindustrial findings (diagnoses, signs, and symptoms) and treatment recommendations* were identified as redundant. The team chose to use *Evaluators clearly distinguish between pre- and postindustrial . . .* as the demanded quality. If the affinity grouping had been assembled into a tree and the tree more carefully analyzed prior to the AHP ranking, this redundancy could have been picked up earlier and the tree modified accordingly. This would undoubtedly have changed some of the AHP scores but probably not the overall order of the results. The on-sight interviews and the ranking took three full workdays, which were spread over a two-week period.

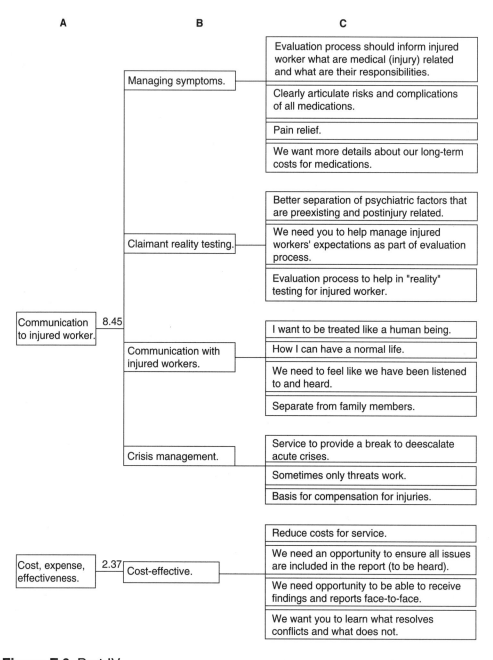

Figure E.3. Part IV

A SURVEY

The eight highest-ranking demanded qualities were used to design a questionnaire with three parts. Part 1 asked customers to rank the importance of each demanded quality from *1 = Does Not Matter* to *5 = Very Strongly Matters.* Part 2 asked them to rank the organization and three competitors from *1 = Poor* to *5 = Excellence* based on their experience of each organization's ability to deliver the demanded qualities. Part 3 was a set of Kano paired questions to ask the customers how they felt if an item was present and how they would feel if it was not present (Figure E.4, Parts 1, 2, and 3).

The raw data for the paired questions is shown in Figure E.5. The number or responses to each question varied slightly as some questions were left blank. The results of Part 1 and Part 2 are shown in the Quality Planning Table (discussion follows).

QUALITY PLANNING TABLE

Results of the survey were entered into a Quality Planning Table (Figure E.6). In this case study, the AHP rankings gathered in the field rather than the results of the customer survey were used to calculate the percentage composite importance ranking. This was done after a debate that emphasized that the AHP ranking had a wider distribution and perhaps more discrimination (12 versus 3) than the rankings of the customer in the field (5 versus 4, highest to lowest). Usually the results of the survey are used as these are captured from a larger number of customers and the sample is more representative of the population of customers as a whole.

Note many of the demanded qualities are compounded phrases, such as, *Evaluations are comprehensive and complete.* Separating this out prior to the affinity grouping and ranking might have uncovered more clarity about what those phrases actually meant to customers.

IDENTIFYING AND RANKING PERFORMANCE MEASURES

When the team first evaluated performance measures with respect to demanded qualities, Row 2, *Reports are both comprehensive and complete,* correlated strongly with all columns, all performance measures. This pattern persisted even after discussion, and the team concluded that the report was perhaps more an indicator of reliability and consistency of the service than a demanded quality, and it was removed to be reconsidered under the reliability deployment. Also note this matrix is more than 50 percent full (Figure E.7).

Figure E.8 shows the results of the Demanded Qualities/Performance Measures Matrix with Row 2 eliminated. The five highest-ranking performance measures plus the performance measure *Including all physicians in evaluation process* were selected by the team and targets agreed to. The latter performance measure was selected even though its overall rating in the matrix was half the next highest-ranking item because data from the paired questions (Figure E.5) suggested it had the potential to distinguish the services and add perceived value to the evaluation process.

FUNCTIONS DEPLOYMENT

The six performance measures were used as input into a Performance Measures/Functions Matrix (Figure E.9), and 11 key functions were identified.

Part 1 Importance. Using a scale where *1 = Does Not Matter and 5 = Very Strongly Matters,* please rate how the following factors influence your decisions when deciding on whom to make a referral to for complex independent evaluations for injured workers.

	Does Not Matter	Somewhat Matters	Matters	Strongly Matters	Very Strongly Matters
A. Previous experience with the comprehensiveness of diagnostic medical evaluations.	1	2	3	4	5
B. Previous experience with comprehensiveness of final reports.	1	2	3	4	5
C. Consistency and completeness in distinguishing preexisting symptoms, findings, and treatments from those directly from the industrial injury.	1	2	3	4	5
D. The level of detail of assessments of current work capacities and/or limitations.	1	2	3	4	5
E. Medical evaluator's direct communication with treating physicians and their ability to have recommendations implemented by treating physician.	1	2	3	4	5
F. Independent medical evaluations are useful to you when challenged during administrative hearings.	1	2	3	4	5
G. Cost of an evaluation.	1	2	3	4	5
H. Medical and legal communities' perception of the medical evaluator's independence from you.	1	2	3	4	5
I. The ability of a layperson to understand important findings and conclusions.	1	2	3	4	5

Figure E.4. Part I

FAILURE MODE DEPLOYMENT

The 11 functions identified were entered into a Functions/Failure Modes Matrix (Figure E.10). Data from the reliability column of the Voice-of-the-Customer Table, Part 2, as well as from the experience of the team as to where the process tended to unravel, were identified and placed into the columns. Two potential failure points were identified to be addressed during new concept deployment.

CREATING AND SELECTING CONCEPTS FOR SERVICE DELIVERY

An adaptation of the process of Concept Selection and Generation developed by Stewart Pugh was used to rank between alternative concepts (Pugh 1991). The Pugh process

Part 2. Based on your experiences, please use the following scale to rate the providers on the items listed.

Scale

1 = *Poor*
2 = *Below Average*
3 = *Average*
4 = *Above Average*
5 = *Excellent*
N = *No Experience with Provider*

	Competitor 1	Competitor 2	Us	Competitor 3
A. Comprehensiveness of the diagnostic medical evaluations.	1 2 3 4 5 N	1 2 3 4 5 N	1 2 3 4 5 N	1 2 3 4 5 N
B. Comprehensiveness of the final reports.	1 2 3 4 5 N	1 2 3 4 5 N	1 2 3 4 5 N	1 2 3 4 5 N
C. Consistency and completeness in distinguishing preexisting symptoms, findings, and treatments from those directly from the industrial injury.	1 2 3 4 5 N	1 2 3 4 5 N	1 2 3 4 5 N	1 2 3 4 5 N
D. The level of detail of assessments of current work capacities and/or limitations.	1 2 3 4 5 N	1 2 3 4 5 N	1 2 3 4 5 N	1 2 3 4 5 N
E. Medical evaluator's direct communication with treating physicians and their ability to have recommendations implemented by treating physician.	1 2 3 4 5 N	1 2 3 4 5 N	1 2 3 4 5 N	1 2 3 4 5 N
F. Independent medical evaluations are useful to you when challenged during administrative hearings.	1 2 3 4 5 N	1 2 3 4 5 N	1 2 3 4 5 N	1 2 3 4 5 N
G. Cost of an evaluation.	1 2 3 4 5 N	1 2 3 4 5 N	1 2 3 4 5 N	1 2 3 4 5 N
H. Medical and legal communities' perception of the medical evaluator's independence from you.	1 2 3 4 5 N	1 2 3 4 5 N	1 2 3 4 5 N	1 2 3 4 5 N
I. The ability of a layperson to understand important findings and conclusions.	1 2 3 4 5 N	1 2 3 4 5 N	1 2 3 4 5 N	1 2 3 4 5 N
J. Overall satisfaction with services.	1 2 3 4 5 N	1 2 3 4 5 N	1 2 3 4 5 N	1 2 3 4 5 N

Figure E.4. Part II

Part 3. This last section asks pairs of multiple-choice questions. Half of the questions ask how you would feel if an item was present; the other half asks how you would feel if the item was not present. Simply select the answer that seems most appropriate for you.

1a. If the diagnostic medical evaluation appears comprehensive, how do you feel?

1. I like it that way.
2. It must be that way.
3. I am neutral.
4. I can live with it that way.
5. I dislike it that way.

1b. If the diagnostic medical evaluation does not seem comprehensive, how do you feel?

1. I like it that way.
2. It must be that way.
3. I am neutral.
4. I can live with it that way.
5. I dislike it that way.

2a. If the final report appears complete and comprehensive, how do you feel?

1. I like it that way.
2. It must be that way.
3. I am neutral.
4. I can live with it that way.
5. I dislike it that way.

2b. If the final report appears less than comprehensive and complete, how do you feel?

1. I like it that way.
2. It must be that way.
3. I am neutral.
4. I can live with it that way.
5. I dislike it that way.

3a. If all the preexisting symptoms, findings, and treatments are clearly distinguished from those associated with the injury, how do you feel?

1. I like it that way.
2. It must be that way.
3. I am neutral.
4. I can live with it that way.
5. I dislike it that way.

3b. If all the preexisting symptoms, findings, and treatments are not clearly distinguished from those related to the industrial injury, how do you feel?

1. I like it that way.
2. It must be that way.
3. I am neutral.
4. I can live with it that way.
5. I dislike it that way.

4a. If there is good detail on the assessments of current work capacities and limitations, how do you feel?

1. I like it that way.
2. It must be that way.
3. I am neutral.
4. I can live with it that way.
5. I dislike it that way.

4b. If there is poor detail on the assessments of current work capacities and limitations, how do you feel?

1. I like it that way.
2. It must be that way.
3. I am neutral.
4. I can live with it that way.
5. I dislike it that way.

Figure E.4. Part III

5a.	If the evaluator directly communicates with the treating physicians and their recommendations are implemented, how do you feel?	1. I like it that way. 2. It must be that way. 3. I am neutral. 4. I can live with it that way. 5. I dislike it that way.
5b.	If the evaluators do not routinely communicate with the treating physicians and their recommendations are not implemented, how do you feel?	1. I like it that way. 2. It must be that way. 3. I am neutral. 4. I can live with it that way. 5. I dislike it that way.
6a.	If the evaluation is very useful to you when challenged during administrative hearings or appeal processes, how to you feel?	1. I like it that way. 2. It must be that way. 3. I am neutral. 4. I can live with it that way. 5. I dislike it that way.
6b.	If the evaluation is of limited usefulness to you when challenged during administrative hearings or appeal processes, how do you feel?	1. I like it that way. 2. It must be that way. 3. I am neutral. 4. I can live with it that way. 5. I dislike it that way.
7a.	If the medical and legal community perceive the evaluator as independent from you, how do you feel?	1. I like it that way. 2. It must be that way. 3. I am neutral. 4. I can live with it that way. 5. I dislike it that way.
7b.	If the medical and legal community do not perceive the evaluator as independent from you, how do you feel?	1. I like it that way. 2. It must be that way. 3. I am neutral. 4. I can live with it that way. 5. I dislike it that way.
8a.	If the findings and conclusions can be understood by a layperson, how do you feel?	1. I like it that way. 2. It must be that way. 3. I am neutral. 4. I can live with it that way. 5. I dislike it that way.
8b.	If some of the findings and conclusions are not readily understandable by a layperson, how do you feel?	1. I like it that way. 2. It must be that way. 3. I am neutral. 4. I can live with it that way. 5. I dislike it that way.

Figure E.4. *Continued.* Part III

1. If the diagnostic medical evaluation appears/does not appear comprehensive and complete, how do you feel?

How do you feel if XX not provided?

How do you feel if XX is provided?	1. I like it that way.	2. It must be that way.	3. I am neutral.	4. I can live with it that way.	5. I dislike it that way.
1. I like it that way.					9
2. It must be that way.					19
3. I am neutral.					3
4. I can live with it that way.					1
5. I dislike it that way.					

2. If the final report appears/does not appear complete and comprehensive, how do you feel?

How do you feel if XX not provided?

How do you feel if XX is provided?	1. I like it that way.	2. It must be that way.	3. I am neutral.	4. I can live with it that way.	5. I dislike it that way.
1. I like it that way.				1	20
2. It must be that way.					9
3. I am neutral.					2
4. I can live with it that way.					
5. I dislike it that way.					

Figure E.5. Part I

3. If all the preexisting symptoms, findings, and treatments are/are not clearly distinguished from those of the injury, how do you feel?

How do you feel if XX not provided?

How do you feel if XX is provided?	1. I like it that way.	2. It must be that way.	3. I am neutral.	4. I can live with it that way.	5. I dislike it that way.
1. I like it that way.					18
2. It must be that way.	1				11
3. I am neutral.					2
4. I can live with it that way.					
5. I dislike it that way.					

4. If there is/is not good detail on the assessments of current work, how do you feel?

How do you feel if XX not provided?

How do you feel if XX is provided?	1. I like it that way.	2. It must be that way.	3. I am neutral.	4. I can live with it that way.	5. I dislike it that way.
1. I like it that way.				3	18
2. It must be that way.					8
3. I am neutral.					2
4. I can live with it that way.					1
5. I dislike it that way.					

Figure E.5. Part II

5. If the evaluators do/do not directly communicate with the treating physicians and their recommendations are not implemented, how do you feel?

How do you feel if XX not provided?

How do you feel if XX is provided?	1. I like it that way.	2. It must be that way.	3. I am neutral.	4. I can live with it that way.	5. I dislike it that way.
1. I like it that way.		2	14	5	3
2. It must be that way.			3		3
3. I am neutral.			1		
4. I can live with it that way.				1	
5. I dislike it that way.					

6. If the evaluation is/is not very useful to you when challenged, how do you feel?

How do you feel if XX not provided?

How do you feel if XX is provided?	1. I like it that way.	2. It must be that way.	3. I am neutral.	4. I can live with it that way.	5. I dislike it that way.
1. I like it that way.				1	19
2. It must be that way.			1		9
3. I am neutral.			1		
4. I can live with it that way.					
5. I dislike it that way.					

Figure E.5. Part III

7. If the medical and legal community perceive/do not perceive the evaluator as being independent from you, how do you feel?

How do you feel if XX not provided?

How do you feel if XX is provided?	1. I like it that way.	2. It must be that way.	3. I am neutral.	4. I can live with it that way.	5. I dislike it that way.
1. I like it that way.	1	3			3
2. It must be that way.			4	2	2
3. I am neutral.		3	6	2	2
4. I can live with it that way.			2		
5. I dislike it that way.					

8. If the findings and conclusions can/cannot be understood by a layperson how do you feel?

How do you feel if XX not provided?

How do you feel if XX is provided?	1. I like it that way.	2. It must be that way.	3. I am neutral.	4. I can live with it that way.	5. I dislike it that way.
1. I like it that way.		1	8	14	3
2. It must be that way.					2
3. I am neutral.			4	2	
4. I can live with it that way.					
5. I dislike it that way.					

Figure E.5. Part IV

Demanded Qualities	Importance AHP Field	Customer Survey Ranking	Our Organization	Competitor 1	Competitor 2	Competitor 3	Target	Ratio of Improvement	Sales Points	DQ Composite Importance	% Composite Importance
1. Diagnostic medical evaluations are comprehensive and complete (i.e., "no surprises later").	12	5	4	4	4	4	4	1	1.5	18	16.2
2. Reports are both comprehensive and complete i.e., "no loose ends".	13	5	4	4	4	4	5	1.25	1.5	23.4	21.1
3. Preexisting factors of impairment and disability are clearly separated from those of injury.	10	5	4	4	4	4	5	1.25	1.5	18.9	17.1
4. Assessments of the current work capacities and limitations are detailed.	12	4	4	4	4	4	5	1.25	1.2	18.5	16.6
5. Recommendations are implemented by workers' treating physicians.	11	4	3	3	3	3	4	1.33	1.2	17.8	16.0
6. Reports withstand challenge during administrative hearings.	6	4	4	3	4	4	4	1	1.2	7.2	6.5
7. You are perceived as independent from the insurer.	4	4	4	3	4	4	4	1	1	4	3.6
8. Findings and conclusions are able to be understood by a layperson.	3	4	4	3	4	4	4	1	1	3	2.7
Weighted Satisfaction			273	260	267	273	319				
Cost		3	4	3	3	3					

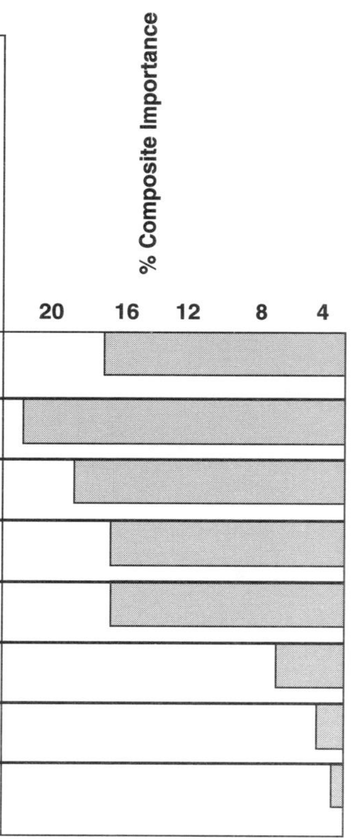

% Composite Importance (chart scale: 20, 16, 12, 8, 4)

Figure E.6.

Demanded Qualities/Performance Measures Matrix

Demanded Qualities	Demanded Quality % Composite Importance	% Symptoms identified	% Findings identified	% Treatments identified	% Opinions and recommendations supported with evidence	% Complete separation of diagnoses, findings, recommendations into industrial versus nonindustrial	% Tasks required in previous job actually tested	% Capacities & impairments quantified or "semiquantified"	% Treating MDs included in the process	% Returned to work	Number of inconsistencies between observers
Direction of Improvement		↑	↑	↑	↑	↑	↑	↑	↑	↑	↓
1. Diagnostic medical evaluations are comprehensive and complete (i.e., no surprises later").	12.00	●	●	◐	○	✓	✓	✓	✓	✓	✓
2. Final reports are both comprehensive and complete.	13.00	●	●	◐	●	●	●	◐	●	●	●
3. Preexisting factors of impairment and disability are clearly separated from those of injury.	10.00	●	✓	✓	●	●	✓	✓	✓	✓	✓
4. Assessments of current work capacities and limitations are detailed.	12.00	✓	○	◐	✓	✓	●	●	✓	✓	●
5. Recommendations are implemented by workers' treating physicians.	11.00	✓	✓	✓	◐	◐	●	✓	●	●	◐
6. Reports withstand challenge during administrative hearings.	6.00	●	◐	✓	●	●	◐	◐	✓	✓	●
7. You are perceived as independent from the insurer.	4.00	◐	✓	●	●	✓	◐	◐	◐	◐	✓
8. Findings and conclusions are able to be understood by a layperson.	3.00	✓	✓	✓	✓	●	✓	◐	✓	✓	◐
Absolute Importance		381.0	225.0	147.0	342.0	321.0	354.0	186.0	228.0	228.0	321.0
Relative Importance		0.138	0.092	0.053	0.124	0.116	0.128	0.067	0.083	0.083	0.116

● Strong Relationship   ◐ Medium Relationship   ○ Weak Relationship   ✓ No Relationship

Figure E.7.

uses paired comparisons with the current industries' best. Several criteria are used and may be weighted. New designs are developed by integrating the best features onto a common platform.

The team generated three concepts to address the failure mode in *Inconsistent findings between different physician observers* to reduce the potential inconsistencies in the report. Each concept included a feedback loop to shape consistency between evaluators into the final report (Figure E.11). The key concept involved a series of phone calls, a series of faxes, or a series of face-to-face meetings between physicians.

Constraints such as organizational time, cycle time, costs, and consistency were chosen as dimensions to evaluate strengths and weaknesses of each of these potential

Demanded Qualities/Performance Measures Matrix	Demanded Quality % Composite Importance	% Symptoms identified	% Findings identified	% Treatments identified	% Opinions and recommendations supported with evidence	% Complete separation of diagnoses, findings, recommendations into industrial versus nonindustrial	% Tasks required in previous job actually tested	% Capacities & impairments quantified or "semiquantified"	% Treating MDs included in the process	% Returned to work	Number of inconsistencies between observers
		Performance Measures									
Direction of Improvement		↑	↑	↑	↑	↑	↑	↑	↑	↑	↓
Demanded Qualities 1. Diagnostic medical evaluations are comprehensive and complete (i.e., no surprises later").	12.00	●	●	◔	○	✓	✓	✓	✓	✓	✓
3. Preexisting factors of impairment and disability are clearly separated from those of injury.	10.00	●	✓	✓	●	●	✓	✓	✓	✓	✓
4. Assessments of current work capacities and limitations are detailed.	12.00	✓	○	◔	✓	✓	●	●	✓	✓	●
5. Recommendations are implemented by workers' treating physicians.	11.00	✓	✓	✓	◔	◔	●	✓	●	●	◔
6. Reports withstand challenge during administrative hearings.	6.00	●	◔	✓	●	●	◔	◔	✓	✓	●
7. You are perceived as independent from the insurer.	4.00	◔	✓	●	●	✓	◔	◔	◔	◔	✓
8. Findings and conclusions are able to be understood by a layperson.	3.00	✓	✓	✓	✓	●	✓	◔	✓	✓	◔
Absolute Importance		264.0	138.0	108.0	225.0	204.0	237.0	147.0	111.0	111.0	204.0
Relative Importance		15.1%	7.9%	6.2%	12.9%	11.7%	13.6%	8.4%	6.3%	6.3%	11.7%
Selected		Y	N	N	Y	Y	Y	N	Y	N	Y
Targets		100			100	100	100		100		0

● Strong Relationship ◔ Medium Relationship ○ Weak Relationship

Figure E.8.

options. First, the team used the AHP process to weight these four constraints. These four constraints and their weightings were then placed into the rows of the New Concepts Selection Matrix. The competing concepts were placed in the columns. Column 2 was chosen as the reference. With this reference point, each of the four constraints for the remaining two concepts are compared as either a + (better), S (same), or – (worse) than the reference concept. These values are placed in the appropriate cell. The reference (Concept 2) rated higher than either Concept 1 (–12) or Concept 3 (–52). It was thus chosen as the design concept for this particular part of the overall service chain.

Performance Measures/ Functions Matrix	Performance Measure Weights	Schedule entire evaluation prior to workers' arrival.	Survey workers prior to arrival.	Survey treating physicians prior to arrival.	Summarize medical records prior to arrival.	Do basic evaluation on all workers.	Summarize and distribute all findings end of day one.	Draft summary initial opinions end of day one.	Do custom work evaluations.	Perform multiple trials of key functional tests.	Use quantitative measures for work evaluations.	Link all opinions to evidence.	Create one summary report.	Check report for internal consistency.	Communicate all findings directly to MDs.	Collect customer satisfaction data at one month.	Collect follow-up outcome data at three months and one year.	Target as %	Units of Measure
% Symptoms identified	15.10	●	◐	◐	◐	◐	◐	●	✓	✓	✓	✓	◐	✓	✓	●	●	100	y/n
% Findings linked to observable data	12.90	✓	◐	◐	✓	✓	◐	◐	●	●	●	●	✓	✓	✓	◐	◐	100	y/n
% Findings separated into industrial or nonindustrial	11.70	◐	●	●	◐	✓	✓	●	✓	✓	✓	◐	●	✓	✓	◐	✓	100	y/n
% Job requirements simulated and tested	13.60	◐	✓	✓	✓	◐	✓	◐	◐	●	◐	◐	◐	✓	✓	◐	✓	100	y/n
% Workers' treating physicians included in process	6.30	●	●	●	✓	✓	✓	✓	✓	✓	✓	✓	✓	✓	●	●	●	100	y/n
Number of unexplained inconsistencies	11.70	●	◐	◐	○	✓	◐	●	◐	◐	◐	◐	●	◐	✓	◐	✓	0	#
Absolute Importance		373.0	281.0	281.0	92.1	86.1	119.0	426.0	192.0	273.0	192.0	227.0	296.0	35.1	56.7	342.0	231.0		
Relative Importance		0.11	0.08	0.08	0.03	0.02	0.03	0.12	0.05	0.08	0.05	0.06	0.08	0.01	0.02	0.10	0.07		
Selected		Y	Y	Y	N	N	N	Y	Y	Y	Y	Y	Y	N	N	Y	Y		

● Strong Relationship ◐ Medium Relationship ○ Weak Relationship

Figure E.9.

TASK DEPLOYMENT

A portion of the Task Deployment Table is shown in Figure E.12.

CLOSING THE LOOP OUTCOME DATA

The organization reported follow-up data at three months and one year on 25 cases (Chaplin et al. 1999). Nineteen (76 percent) of the workers were determined to have received maximal medical treatment. For this group, residual impairments were defined and recommendations made with regard to vocational retraining. Further treatment was recommended for the remaining six (24 percent). Follow-up data at three months indicated that nine (47 percent) of the 19 cases for which a determination was made that the injured worker had reached maximal medical improvement had findings that were immediately accepted by the worker, his or her attorney, and the insurer. The remaining 10 workers elected to enter into an appeal process. Follow-up at one year indicated that three additional cases were settled without appeal, and two persons had appeal hearings

Functions/Failure Modes Matrix		Weight of Functions	Failure Modes					
			Incomplete evaluations, workers not completing requested activities	Having to add additional procedures & tests during evaluation period	Failure of team to adapt to unforeseen circumstances	Breakdown in team following policies and procedures	After evaluation period, discover some critical tasks are incomplete	Inconsistent findings between different physician evaluators
Functions	Schedule entire evaluation prior to workers' arrival.	10.7	●	◕	✓	●	✓	✓
	Survey workers prior to arrival.	8.00	●	✓	◕	◕	✓	◕
	Survey treating physician prior to arrival.	8.00	✓	●	◕	◕	✓	◕
	Draft summary initial opinions by the end of day one.	12.2	✓	●	◕	✓	◕	●
	Do custom work evaluations.	5.50	●	✓	✓	✓	◕	○
	Perform multiple trials of key functional tests.	7.80	✓	✓	✓	✓	◕	○
	Use quantitative measures for work evaluations.	5.50	✓	✓	✓	◕	◕	✓
	Link all opinions to evidence.	6.50	✓	✓	✓	✓	◕	◕
	Create one summary report.	8.50	✓	○	✓	✓	✓	●
	Collect customer satisfaction data at one month.	9.80	●	✓	✓	✓	●	●
	Collect follow-up outcome data at three months and one year.	6.60	✓	✓	✓	✓	◕	✓
Absolute Importance			306.	222.	84.6	160.	220.	355.
Relative Importance			22.7%	16.5%	6.3%	11.9%	16.3%	26.3%
Selected			Y	N	N	N	N	Y

● Strong Relationship   ◕ Medium Relationship   ○ Weak Relationship

Figure E.10.

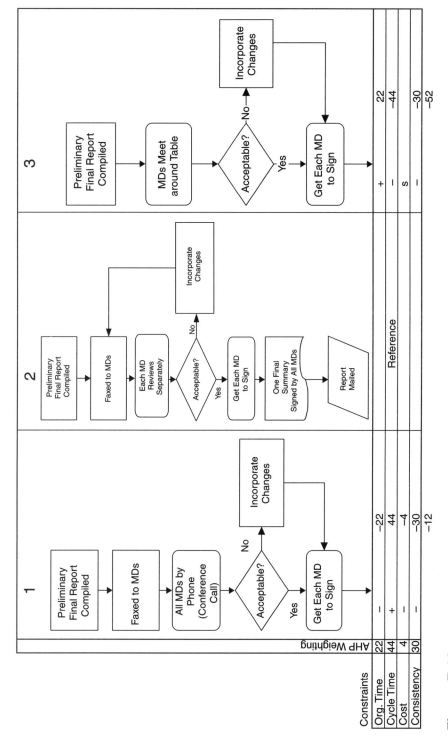

Figure E.11.

281

Task Deployment Table

What	Who	When	Where	How	How Much	Why	Other
All planning and preadmit scheduling complete.	Marketing Secretary	Start 3 weeks prior to planned admit. Complete 5 days before	CRHSD	Phone and Fax		Build template for evaluation.	
Send and collect preadmit scheduling patient questionnaire.	Marketing Secretary	Send 2 weeks before planned admit.	CRHSD	Mail Phone		Build complete list of symptoms and impairments.	
Send questionnaire and make call to treating physician.	Marketing Secretary Managing MD Peer to Peer	Survey 2 weeks. Call 1 week.	CRHSD	Mail Phone		Build complete list of symptoms, diagnoses, and impairments.	
Working summary completed at end of day 1.	Managing MD	Day 1.	CRHSD	Dictation		Get everyone on same page.	
First notification to evaluators when reports late.	Marketing Secretary	Next working day after due date.	At MDs office	Phone and Fax		Feedback to keep commitments.	
Third notification if report is late.	Managing MD Peer to Peer	If misses deadline by 1 week or misses 3 deadlines in a row.	At MDs office	Phone		Feedback to keep commitments or or change commitments.	

Figure E.12.

in which the rulings upheld the completeness of the evaluation process and its accuracy and the cases were closed. Two persons are still awaiting appeal hearings, one person died of myocardial infarction unrelated to his work injury, and one case has been lost to follow-up.

As presented earlier, over our five-year experience with this same customer base, we averaged 22 (±4) evaluations per year. The QFD project started with interviews in the field in August 1997, and the implementation of the new system occurred in November of 1997. Formal and informal feedback from customers since implementation was extremely positive. During 1998, the facility had evaluated 50 injured workers, a referral rate that is slightly more than double that of the average volume for past years.

The interviews were conducted in the field in August of 1997, and, subsequently, the team met on a weekly basis to work on the QFD process. Three-and-one-half months elapsed between the initial meeting and the deployment of changes.

Appendix F

QFD Healthcare Case Study

Emergency Department: Remodeling and Design

by James Bruer[1]

THE SITUATION

The Emergency Department of New England Memorial Hospital lacked sufficient space to meet current code requirements and provide for patient privacy, physician sleeping areas, and family waiting rooms. There was no separate entrance for patients arriving by ambulance and ambulatory walk-ins. The Board of Trustees requested that a plan for renovation of the facility be drafted and a fund-raising campaign initiated to finance the eventual construction. The hospital construction manager was commissioned to coordinate the project. A project architect was retained, and work was begun in the traditional fashion with the architect meeting with physicians, maintenance, and department staff. After 3 to 4 weeks, rumblings of dissatisfaction and concern were being heard throughout the ranks. It was feared that the critical needs of support departments, staff, and non-departmental physicians would not be met; the project began to lag behind its timetable. Apart from the actual construction, the project was going to require unified support across the institution. The assistant vice president in charge of the maintenance areas requested assistance in putting the project back on track.

THE APPLICATION

This is one of those QFD applications that used zero matrices. The process was driven by a deep commitment to gather the voice of the customer. This commitment was natural because the team was the customer. Thus, this case is really QFD thinking passed on to the supplier who knew nothing about QFD.

Since the root cause of people's dissatisfaction was a feeling that their needs were not being met, it was decided to "listen to the voice of the customer" through a "blitz" QFD process. Managers and physicians from all affected departments (about 20 in all) were requested to participate in two 4-hour sessions on two consecutive days. A professional QFD consultant was retained to present the QFD philosophy and approach

[1]James Bruer was the Vice President of Operations for New England Memorial Hospital from 1988 to 1994. In 1990 James became excited about the power of QFD. Summaries of the two cases presented here, cases F and G represent some of the earliest applications of QFD to the healthcare environment.

285

during the first session and to begin to elicit "needs" from the participants. The design architect and a management engineer from a healthcare consultanting firm with experience in emergency department design were also asked to attend. The management engineer was there to lend credibility to the process, should anyone question its viability, and to rescue the situation if it looked as if things were not going well. In the end, his sole comment was "I've never seen a design process work so effectively." Each of the members of the group was asked to state their needs, wishes, and desires if the ideal department could be designed; others were free to comment and clarify what they were hearing. Understanding between the parties grew at a rapid pace. The construction manager took meticulous notes and produced a document that was turned over to the architect at the end of the sessions. The cover sheet had

> Main Themes to Ponder
> Minimize: Time Spent per Patient Visit
> > Real Time
> > Perceived Time
> Maximize: Clinical Efficiency
> > Nurses Do Nursing
> > Others Do Other Stuff
> Realize: Logistics of Service
> > 24 Hours
> > 7 Days a Week
> Conceptualize: Voice of the Future
> > Plan Ahead
> > Keep the Plan Flexible
> Prioritize: Patient Care
> > Hospital-Wide Standard

This was followed by further consideration of communications, supplies, admittings, turnaround times, and security. The body of the document stated the need of 32 customers from two perspectives, the systems and the physical requirements. Both of these were further broken down from the perspective of each of the 32 customer segments and the Emergency Department. Sometimes there were action and/or solutions provided.

The following were the needs of the Environmental Services department. This was a broader responsibility than just cleaning. Their needs included

Systems Requirements
To be able to provide 24-hour service
Control the distribution of linens to ambulance services
Effective recycling
Discreet removal of trash
Efficient thorough cleaning

Physical Requirments	**Solutions**
Easy-to-clean rooms	Hanging base cabinets
	No tile floors
	Smooth walls
	And so on

The Emergency Department wanted a 5-minute response to spills, a sterile supply, no-slip floors, and more. In the document, it is clear that needs, solutions, problems, and so on are all intermingled.

THE RESULTS

While not "pure" QFD, this rudimentary approach yielded wonderful results. The team continued to meet from time to time as the architect brought in various drawings based on the earlier input. Each was critiqued on the basis of the Needs Document, and input to fine-tune the design was given. Everyone felt (for good reason), that they were included in the process. The remodeling project was limited to a smaller area than was generally felt needed to properly accommodate the necessary functions. In the end, everything fit, the various systems worked well together, and patients were pleased to receive treatment in the facility. The project was completed on time and within budget.

THINGS LEARNED

QFD does not have to be stringent or rigid; it is important to capture the philosophy or essence of the process first and apply it, striving for mastery as you continue to learn project by project, step by step. In retrospect, the team members could see how more time spent in "working through the matrices" could have yielded even greater results. If a decision to use QFD had been made up front, some of the initial frustration at the project's beginning would have been avoided. The project architect was appreciative of the process but at times felt uncomfortable because he was not in control; the customer was. What normally would be a finished design became a living document as the architect received new feedback on how he missed the mark. The team review process was more rigorous than usual. Out of courtesy to his firm, the facilities requirement for this type of design process should have been included in the original RFP for services. A requirement for the project leader to attend a QFD seminar would have been a reasonable expectation.

Just last week, the former head of the Emergency Room and the former head of Nursing both said it was the best design project they had ever worked in.

Appendix G

QFD Healthcare Case Study

Rehab Concepts: Service Line Development

by James Bruer

THE SITUATION

In 1990, hospitals across the country were looking for new services in which market niches could be developed to expand their revenue base. New England Memorial Hospital in Stoneham, Massachusetts, had a strong outpatient rehabilitation program and sought to build on that strength by entering the occupational medicine market. A Performa Budget plan was constructed based on existing patient volumes and projections of new business. Executive management decided to approve funds and moved forward with the leasing of space for an off-campus, free-standing facility. Two board-certified physicians were interested in providing the medical leadership of the program; therapists from the existing department and a program manager from one of the physicians' practices were retained, equipment was ordered, and operations began.

During the initial start-up phase, as the first patients were entering the program, concerns emerged that something was not "right" with the program. The enthusiasm of the start-up and very quick launch was fading into the reality of making a program succeed. Management began to be concerned that a more effective planning process should have been put in place. Since several hospital managers had recently received training in QFD and were looking for an opportunity to try out the new quality tool, it was decided to do a prototype using the rehabilitation program. A project team consisting of the physician, manager, therapists, support personnel, and the hospital planner was formed. Four-hour sessions were scheduled over three consecutive days.

THE APPLICATION

Three team meetings were planned. At the first, a long list of staff-constructed customer needs was presented. The list was mixed with solutions, needs, and measures—it was large and unwieldy; more importantly, it was obviously unfocused. The matrix had 128 demanded qualities with one to four levels of detail. The matrix also had 138 performance measures with one to four levels of detail. The facilitator suggested that the team members prioritize the list by cutting and pasting each "customer need." The result was eight needs. At this point, the most important need was *Return to Work*. The facilitator was surprised with this result. When asked whom this represented, the staff answered the insurance company and the employer because the patient did not pay the bill. After a short break and talking to several patients in therapy on location, the most important need became *Resume Normal Lifestyle.* This was two times more important than *Return to Work.* The original eight needs representing the employer and the insurance company were integrated with the patients' need to start the Demanded Qualities/Performance Measures Matrix (Figure G.1).

While the team struggled in refining customer needs, defining things that needed to be controlled or measured, "quality characteristics" seemed to be a bigger challenge. It seemed as if a metric was emerging where none had existed before; the concept of "measurement for results" or benchmarking was pushing itself forward with some resistance. While budgetary performance was routinely measured, the "qualitative" aspects of the care process rarely were; things were "OK" if no one was complaining, and the complaints people worried about came from physicians. Measurables were difficult to think about clearly, and the team did not want to. The facilitator had to push us along.

Our rather simple Demanded Qualities/Performance Measures Matrix was beginning to take on final form. The "fill-in-the-blanks" phase of determining strength of relationships between needs and performance measures looked at first to be a 5-minute project—it was not. The process of *thinking* about each relationship revealed differences in opinion about the *meanings* of the words that we had chosen. A glossary would have been helpful. We were also being forced to think nonlinearly, and *new* needs and characteristics not thought of before jumped out at the team.

With the core matrix, complete attention turned to listing important competitors and determining performance targets for the customer needs and quality characteristics. Management was impressed with detailed knowledge the staff had of competing programs; it was much better than anticipated and prompted thoughts of, "if only we had known." The information, if available earlier, may have had an impact on choosing the site location or whether to enter the market at all. The list of competitors was longer than anyone had anticipated. Just seeing them listed on one sheet along with their relative strengths gave one a sense of urgency to get things moving.

THE RESULTS

The program was brought into clearer focus. The strength and need for the program were in the concentrated rehabilitation of recuperating employees as opposed to "work hardening." To be successful, the patient's need to be able to function as before the injury must be met. The reputation of the service would be built on positive patient outcomes as defined by the ability of the patient to resume "activities of daily living." The patient—as opposed to the employer and insurer—became the primary customer and program focus. Yes, this should have been obvious initially; however, the desire for marketshare and a diversified revenue stream for the hospital had clouded the true vision of patient service and confused the program objective—patient wellness. The team was surprised to find that location, transportation, and professional accomplishments of staff were not the leading "needs" of the patients but rather represented "Performance Measures" patients desired. In this intensely personal recovery program, forming constructive relationships between patient and provider was essential. The QFD project revealed that the relationships between staff served as a model for this. It became equally clear that a common treatment philosophy was needed for staff relationships to be effective. Here a major

Rehab Concepts

Legend:
- ● Strong Relationship
- ◑ Medium Relationship
- ○ Weak Relationship
- ⊙ Strong Positive
- ○ Positive
- ※ Negative
- × Strong Negative

Demanded Quality (right-side assessment)

Category	Demanded Quality	Customer Importance	Us	Them 1	Them 2	Them 3	Them 4	Them 5	Target	Ratio of Improvement	Sales Point	DQ Composite Importance	% Composite Importance
Effective Communication	Clear Instructions	1.60	4	4	3	3	3	3	5	1.25	1	2.00	0.01
Effective Communication	Rehab Team Works Together	7.44	2	4	3	2	3	2	5	2.50	1	18.60	0.07
Restorative Treatment	Treatment Clear	2.88	4	4	3	3	3	3	4	1.00	1	2.88	0.01
Restorative Treatment	Return to Work	17.00	3	4	3	3	4	3	5	1.67	2	56.67	0.21
Restorative Treatment	Resume Normal Lifestyle	32.90	2	3	3	2	4	3	4	2.00	2	131.60	0.50
Restorative Treatment	Get in Shape	5.49	3	4	3	3	3	3	4	1.33	1	7.32	0.03
Restorative Treatment	Prevent Reoccurrence	5.49	3	4	3	3	4	3	5	1.67	2	18.30	0.07
Emotional Support	Nice Physical Environment	14.40	4	4	2	3	3	3	4	1.00	1	14.40	0.05
Emotional Support	Interpersonal Support	1.60	3	3	3	3	3	3	4	1.33	1	2.13	0.01
Hassle Free Services	Easy Paperwork	2.20	4	4	4	3	3	4	5	1.25	1	2.75	0.01
Hassle Free Services	Easy Access to Facility	3.00	4	3	4	4	3	3	4	1.00	1	3.00	0.01
Hassle Free Services	Easy Access to Services	1.32	4	3	4	3	3	4	4	1.00	1	1.32	0.00
Hassle Free Services	Equipment Available	4.40	5	3	4	4	3	3	5	1.00	1	4.40	0.02

Performance Level (technical measures — bottom summary)

Category	Measure	Absolute Importance	Relative Importance	Target
Measure Clarity	Rehab Concept	44.94	0.6%	4
Measure Clarity	# of Reinstructions	108.93	1.4%	4
Measure Clarity	# of Communications in File	495.94	6.2%	4
Measure Clarity	% Independent Exercise Correct	670.94	8.4%	4
Fix the Patient	# of Days out of Work	1081.65	13.5%	4
Fix the Patient	# of Days to Full Duty	970.80	12.1%	4
Fix the Patient	% Normal Activity Returned	1763.16	22.0%	4
Fix the Patient	Biomechanical Meas. Before/After	309.05	3.9%	4
Fix the Patient	Time to Reoccurrence	348.16	4.3%	5
Emotional Support	Defined Personal Space	266.21	3.3%	4
Emotional Support	# of Air Exchangers	14.40	0.2%	4
Emotional Support	# of Lumins	14.40	0.2%	5
Emotional Support	% Items in Place	151.80	1.9%	5
Emotional Support	Sq. Ft/Person	132.60	1.7%	4
Hassle-Free	Staff Min on No-Physical Issues	356.38	4.5%	5
Hassle-Free	# Minutes to Complete	24.75	0.3%	5
Hassle-Free	Complexity Measure	24.75	0.3%	5
Hassle-Free	% Answers Used	24.75	0.3%	4
Hassle-Free	# of Late Appointments/Commuting	3.00	0.0%	4
Hassle-Free	# Days from Ref. to Initial Treat.	483.63	6.0%	5
Hassle-Free	# of Calls to Complete Regist.	127.10	0.5%	5
Hassle-Free	% Time Waiting for Equipment	39.60	0.5%	4
Hassle-Free	% Downtime of Equipment	550.92	6.9%	5

Figure G.1.

problem became evident: The therapists had been trained in two different treatment philosophies and were adamant concerning their individual approaches. The QFD exercise had revealed that the service was in conflict over how to deliver care. Sadly, efforts to solve this problem eventually led one of the staff members to resign in frustration, and valuable time was lost in moving the program forward. A positive outcome was that program participants were routinely asked about their needs and desires—it became a part of the culture almost overnight.

THINGS LEARNED

QFD works very well as a service line planning tool for both new services and existing services that need improvement in quality, cost, and customer service. QFD can be used effectively as a *first step* in writing the business plan, development of outlines for operational policies, and regulatory compliance programs for complex medical services. Most importantly, it can lead you to gain deeper understanding of the culture and environment in which you are operating and its importance as a cornerstone of any enterprise. While QFD was useful in remediation of existing problems, earlier use of the tool may have prevented flaws in the program design that limited its long-term success. Healthcare as an industry is not particularly used to the detailed design and development discipline one finds in general industry. Decisions are often in a top-down, crisis management mode. In clinical situations, quick decision making based on experience, without undo "analysis," is placed at a premium. If the doctor and patient need or want something, it must be done NOW! Using QFD as a business-planning tool naturally challenges this culture, resulting in early success (experiencing some *aha*s) and strong follow-through.

Appendix H

Healthcare and Healthcare–Related Articles

The Articles Cited Below Were Published in the Transactions from Symposia on Quality Function Deployment.[1]

Prepared by Joe A. Miller

Number 1/ 1989

Article C. *QFD in the Development of a New Medical Device,* Jose R. Rodriguez-Soria, Ernst & Whinney.

Healthcare Company: The Kendall Company (ASSUMED)

Abstract: A healthcare products company, implementing Quality Improvement based on *prevention* and *improvement* for two years, elected to pilot QFD on a development project already underway. The company was developing a new device for treating vascular disorders by compression with its conventional development approaches. QFD was introduced to the team by a brief overview. Specific tools were taught as needed. Marketing leadership in the QFD process was established early. Realizing the need to more clearly define the "customer" lead to study of market segmentation and structure. The team conducted customer interviews, focus groups, and an open-ended assessment of "needs." A House of Quality was constructed and analyzed, reducing 72 customer requirements to 24 and 123 product requirements to 28. The QFD study results were deemed extremely helpful in understanding the market and in the design and development of the product.

[1]Quality Function Deployment Institute
1140 Morehead Ct.
Ann Arbor, Mich. 48103-6181 USA
Electronic mail General Information: information@qfdi.org
Webmaster: qfdi@qfdi.org

Number 2/1990

> *The Application of QFD for a Hospital-Controlled Substance System,* P. Harwood, University of California—Irvine Medical Center; J. Naughton, Expert Knowledge Systems.

Article H. *Introducing QFD into an Organization,* Robert Stoy, Dennis McDonald, Beckman Industries, Inc., and James Naughton, Expert Knowledge Systems.

Healthcare Company: Beckman Instruments, Diagnostic Systems Group

Abstract: Piloting QFD on a new product definition, Beckman Instruments Diagnostics Systems Group sought to provide a supportive environment and assure project success. Beckman established a middle-management "support team" to provide resources and an organizational focus for the core technical project team using QFD, and to learn the QFD process itself. The support team helped identify and set "boundaries" for the core QFD team. These boundaries, and the process of establishing and reviewing them, helped clarify company goals for the team, clarified team and management expectations, and provided a valuable means of communication between the team and executive management.

Article W. *Incorporating Market Research into the Product-Development Process,* Tanya L. Domke, GE Medical Systems.

Healthcare Company: GE Medical Systems

Abstract: A product-development team at GE gained strength by organizing cross-functionally. Following QFD as a structured design process, marketing research was used to assure customer involvement. The QFD "House of Quality" provided the structure and *customer* focus. Market research helped define the Demanded Quality component of the house and provided the *customer* focus. The market research methods used included personal interviews with customers and a technique called "SIMALTO"—Simultaneous Multi-Attribute Level Trade-Off. This technique allowed the team to survey many individuals through personal interviews yet gain quantitative data. Participants played a game simulating the purchase process. The results became a dynamic market model that determined feature and price trade-offs, market segmentation, and competitive assessment.

Number 3/1991

Article 22. *The Strategic Approach to Market Research,* D. A. Ginder, Mech Group, Inc.; N. Donforio, GE Medical Systems.

Healthcare Company: GE Medical Systems

Abstract: An approach to planning and managing Market Research is proposed and illustrated. The method consists of systematically using company goals to identify which (geographic) market segments can best support those goals, identifying which customer types in those important segments are most important and how to approach them. The actual focus group collection of requirements from those customers most important to the company's success is described. Key questions "What do you really want" and "why do you want that" can be utilized to determine *expected, requested,* and *inferred* requirements. QFD Matrix analysis methods and rating methods that support this approach are described and illustrated. The technique includes volume/revenue estimates and a customer importance weight method that has been successfully used by such companies as JI Case, Harley-Davidson Motor Co., 3M Corp., and many smaller companies.

Article 30. *Patient Designed Hospital Care: An Oxymoron No Longer,*
  L. E. Kelly, Medical Center of Central Massachusetts.

Number 4/1992

Article 5. *How QFD Saved a Company—The Renaissance Spirometry System,* O. Kaelin, Puritan Bennett Company, Boston Division, and R. L. Klein, Applied Marketing Science, Inc.

Healthcare Company: Puritan Bennett Company, Boston Division

Abstract: The Boston Division of Puritan Bennett makes spirometers, devices used by doctors to measure lung function and detect pulmonary disease. In a competitive market of over 20 manufacturers, PB was a market leader with over 15 percent of the market. In the summer of 1990, they faced a crisis. A major new competitor had introduced a new product priced at half of their product's current price. This was less than Puritan Bennett's product cost to make. The sales and market share of their existing product fell precipitously. Management was faced with the task of either developing a competitive response or shutting down. They chose to stay and fight and used QFD to develop a product that would meet this threat.

In September 1991, the Boston Division introduced their sales force to the result of their development effort. Their new spirometer was designed to respond to the Voice of the Customer and is priced below their competitor's product. Market response has been overwhelming.

This presentation will describe in detail how a small company (25 people) identified the Voice of the Customer, linked it to engineering characteristics, and then used that information to guide the development of the product that has saved the company.

Article 22. *Multiphase QFD Studies for Product and Services Development,*
  Joe A. Miller, The Focus Consulting Group, Inc., and Armando Bombino, Baxter Healthcare Corporation.

Healthcare Company: Baxter Healthcare Corporation

Abstract: Quality Function Deployment is a structured component of a Customer-Satisfaction driven Total Quality Management (TQM) process. It helps link the basic concepts of TQM into the product and service development processes. Training cross-functional product or service development teams in multiple phase applications of QFD enabled critical decisions by providing critical information needs earlier in the development cycle. This was accomplished by rapid developing of all the QFD matrices pertinent to the full cycle from concept through product introduction. QFD training and team facilitation methods and chart development techniques deliberately kept flexible are applicable to a wide variety of project needs. QFD has been used in a range of applications from new development projects to maintenance of current products and services.

Article 28. *Hospital Marketing's Role in TQI; QFD,* Duane Koller, Meadville Medical Center.

Healthcare Institution: Meadville Medical Center, Meadville, Penn

Abstract: As part of their Total Quality Improvement (TQI) program, the Meadville Medical Center linked the marketing function more closely to operations through development of a research system using the Quality Function Development (sic) tool. This paper examines their experience of melding qualitative and quantitative market research with the development of a QFD A1 matrix. The linkage of existing market research programs with a QFD matrix yielded improved quality of customer research and improved acceptance of the output.

5/1993

Article 1. *Market Expansion Analysis Through QFD,* J. A. Miller, Quality Processing Consulting, and H. N. Tucker, Clintec Nutrition.

Healthcare Company: Clintec Nutrition Company

Abstract: This report presents the approach and findings from a House-of-Quality–based analysis of how to cause expansion of the entire clinical nutrition business worldwide. Clinical nutrition had been shown to have beneficial effect on clinical outcomes and significant potential for reducing overall healthcare costs, but the market response did not always seem to recognize these benefits. The analysis sought to identify why and was based on specific business expansion.

A progressive analysis of the two major areas in this marketplace, enterals and parenterals, separately identified key market segments and then the key customers, beneficiaries, and decision makers within those segments. The wants, needs, and leverage factors important to those "Customers" were identified and prioritized for each market and were then consolidated into a market-wide priority. Approaches to address these wants and needs were identified, including several existing activities. For key approaches, a brief statement framing improvement opportunities and simple measures of progress were drafted. Existing or proposed specific initiatives were compared to the key approaches identified for business expansion and prioritized based on the importance of the approaches.

Article 34. *Applying QFD to Healthcare Services: A Case Study at the University of Michigan Medical Center,* D. M. Ehrlich, Ph.D., and D. J. Hertz, University of Michigan Medical Center.

Healthcare Institution: University of Michigan Medical Center

Revised Abstract: This is an interim report of how The University of Michigan Medical Center (UMMC) piloted Quality Function Deployment (QFD) in a new unit consolidating several separated diagnostic procedures into one unit. Based upon early TQM successes, the organization employed QFD VOC analysis to realign resources to meet valid customer requirements of the combined groups in order to stimulate service volume by better satisfying customer desires. The article discusses the UMMC QFD approach, articulates experiences learned, identifies changes that have been implemented, quantifies the financial benefits that have resulted from those changes, and offers ideas on how best to utilize QFD at a referral hospital.

Number 6/1994

Article 15. *Additional Applications for QFD Matrices,* A. E. Uber, III, and D. L. Gigler, Medrad, Inc.

Healthcare Company: Medrad, Inc.

Abstract: Medrad, Inc., a provider of imaging products, successfully utilized Mind Mapping, experiment design sheets, and a QFD House of Quality matrix format to relate electromechanical system parts to phenomena, and phenomena to phenomena for a film changer machine improvement initiative Medrad's senior managers also utilized a QFD matrix analysis to help select combinations of projects that could best provide for employee, end user, and stockholder goals. This process provided a basis for extensive and valuable discussion of proposed programs.

Article 26. *Applying Quality Function Deployment in Healthcare Services: The Princeton Foot Clinic,* J. Gibson, Baptist Health System.

Healthcare Institution: Princeton Foot Clinic, Princeton Baptist Medical Center

Revised Abstract: The Princeton Foot Clinic sought market differentiation through QFD in the face of competition, economic pressures, and healthcare reform. The initiative utilized Organizational deployment, and Voice of the Customer (VOCT) deployment; together with Quality, Reliability, Function, and Process deployments in a C-A-P-D process. A multifunctional task force confirmed the importance of timeliness, convenience, and courtesy, and discovered items such as referral flexibility and procedure explanation. Identification of key functions, failure points, and processes helped plan a new PFC concept and do what was necessary to prepare for getting the PFC off the ground.

Article 27. *Designing The Voice of the Customer into a New Hospital Surgery Center,* S. Macfarlane and K. Eager, The Quality Advisor, Inc.

Healthcare Institution: Kennewick General Hospital, Kennewick, Wash.

Abstract: In a changing healthcare environment, small free-standing facilities are competing with hospital operating rooms for surgery business. Hospitals, to get into the act, are building "surgery centers" that "feel" unattached, yet still benefit from the hospital's vast resources. Kennewick General Hospital saw that if they did not get competitive against the free-standing facilities, they would not be in the surgery business. Their challenge was to *change* the process by which hospitals and their employees provide care in an efficient, customer-oriented way.

A cross-functional team of hospital employees, using Quality Function Deployment to design the surgery process for their new surgery center, conducted focus group meetings to determine Customers' Requirements, followed by surveys to the same customer groups, which included Patients and Patient Families, Physicians, and Physician Office Staff. This paper describes what worked and what did not when it came to defining customer requirements and the new surgery process. It outlines a methodology, not restricted to healthcare, for defining customer requirements as well as specific recommendations for hospitals wanting to remain competitive.

Article 28. *Cardiac Arrest! QFD on the Heart and Soul of a Medical Center,* V. Alterescu, D. Newhart, and F. Tiedemann, John Muir Medical Center.

Healthcare Institution: John Muir Medical Center

Abstract: John Muir Medical Center conducted QFD projects in three clinical service areas; Cardiology, Oncology, and Rehabilitation, each an area undergoing radical change due to governmental and marketplace reform, and also as a result of serious competitor threats. The success of each project was directly related to the amount of experience the organization had sequentially developed in using the process. Cardiology resulted in a virtual agreement to disband without consensus, oncology resulted in very specific recommendations for a breast cancer program, and rehabilitation in a comprehensive overview of future direction and product design. The existence of interdisciplinary teams focused on developing services systematically tied to customer desires was as unique for John Muir Medical Center (JMMC) as for many other acute care hospitals. Since the provision of health services is in part dominated by physicians, a large vested group of internal customers, and in the past, success was essentially a matter of attracting physicians, QFD has become particularly apt since one of its strengths is the prioritization of customer wants. Had QFD not been done for these projects, the organization would have attempted a very different set of services built around the voice of a single internal customer.

The themes common to these projects indicate certain issues about the use of QFD in a healthcare setting. The critical success factors applicable to QFD at John Muir Medical Center were: (1) carefully designed group dynamics, (2) appropriate complexity of the project, (3) overall quality of facilitation and chairmanship, (4) manner in which the VOC was performed, (5) relationship between the working QFD group and key stakeholders, and (6) comprehensive training in QFD.

Article 29. *QFD in Healthcare: Identifying Methods to Tailor QFD to a Service Industry. A Case Study at the University Of Michigan Medical Center,* D. Ehrlich and E. Kratochwill, University of Michigan Medical Center.

Healthcare Institution: University of Michigan Medical Center

Abstract: The University of Michigan Medical Center (UMMC) piloted Quality Function Deployment (QFD) in a new unit that consolidated several diagnostic procedures into one unit. The objective was to learn when QFD is most appropriate for a hospital and to stimulate service volume at the new unit. An interim review was presented at the 5th Annual QFD Symposium. At the time of this report, the team had nearly completed the study and written a summary paper describing when and how QFD is most applicable at a large healthcare organization. This session will discuss four issues: (1) the UMMC QFD approach, which included implementing changes as information was obtained; (2) the difficulties experienced in applying QFD to healthcare, such as how to obtain and benchmark intangible competitor data; (3) the benefits derived from QFD (for both the unit and the entire organization); and (4) the ways to tailor QFD to healthcare and the service sector.

Number 7/1995

Article 9. *QFD Robust Design and Professional Services: Hospital Emergency Room Case,* S. Macfarlane and K. Eager, Black Sheep Engineering Services.

Healthcare Institution: NOT DISCLOSED

Abstract: A new application of Robust Design Methods; this study challenges the paradigm that Robust Design does not apply to a service or social science. A simple Robust Design approach was used to optimize the process of a hospital emergency room. Average patient length of stay (LOS) was selected as a key quality characteristic from a simplified QFD. Results show a reduction in (LOS) of 25 percent without major capital investment for an expanded facility. Confirmation runs showed excellent repeatability. The greatest challenge was helping the team accept and implement the results, thus improving quality without larger staffs, facilities, and budgets. This study suggests that Robust Design Methods can be used to optimize processes outside the product-development arena.

Article 10. *Happy Feet, Part II: The Return of the Princeton Foot Clinic—or— The QFD Viral Strategy,* J. Gibson, Baptist Health System.

Healthcare Institution: Princeton Foot Clinic, Baptist Health System

Abstract: The Princeton Foot Clinic is a hospital-based foot treatment service developed using QFD principles to identify the spoken and unspoken needs of customers, including comprehensive patient self-care and timely follow-up on patient outcomes to referring physicians. QFD results enabled the clinic to overcome political hurdles involving location of the service. When ultimately the need to have access to technology without duplicating equipment meant reintegrating the clinic into the hospital's rehabilitation services, information and procedures derived from the QFD process had a positive "viral" impact on the larger organization. The use of QFD has resulted in greater awareness of the customer among all parties involved with the clinic and has strengthened the customer focus in the larger rehabilitation services and the entire out-patient scheduling system.

Article 11. *Reconciling Different Customer Needs,* Ian Ferguson, Ian Ferguson Associates.

Healthcare Institution/Company: Not Specified

Abstract: Using an Influenza drug, the Insertion of an Arterial Catheter, and an Asthma Inhaler for examples, the differences of importance of needs and features to different members of a customer supplier chain are examined. These differing features can often require what would appear to be conflicting values for the Product to have high evaluation to the various "Customers." A two-stage mechanism is described that evaluates the design features at each level of deployment by linking the relative level needs, enabling a rational choice of values to be made at each level that will result in high satisfaction at each level of Customer. The mechanisms employed are illustrated by detailed examples.

Number 8/1996

Article 7. **"QFD** *Implementation in Hospital Housekeeping Services"—TQM in CBM Co., Ltd.,* Noriharu Kaneko, Service Quality Management Ltd. (Japan).

Healthcare Company/Institution: Chubu Building Maintenance Co., Ltd. and several unspecified hospitals

Abstract: CBU Co., Ltd., provides contract hospital housekeeping services. One of the greatest threats to patient health is infectious disease. Hospitals must go to great lengths to see that disease does not spread from one patient to the next. Mr. Kaneko, one of the first to apply QFD to services, shows how his company utilized QFD to identify their customer's Required Quality and develop standard procedures and Handbooks and Administrative Function Deployment Charts. ISO9000 compliance to assure cleaning crews do the job right the first time resulted in ISO 9002 Certification.

Article 8. *A Customer-Integrated Decision-Making/QFD Project (CIDM/QFD) by a Multifunction Team of Healthcare Providers*

Planning a Treatment System for Adults with Attention Deficit Disorder (ADD), Douglas W. Pentz, Ph.D., Judith Daniels, M.D., Thomas E. D'Erminio, LISW, B.C., and Bill Barnard, BS.CS, CPIM.

Healthcare Institution/Company: Not Specified

Abstract: This paper describes the development of a treatment system for adults with Attention Deficit Disorder (ADD). The objective of the study was an understanding of the strategic issues of this system and their priorities. The project team was a multi-function team of healthcare professionals using a process called Customer-Integrated Decision-Making/Quality Function Deployment (CIDM/QFD). The effort began in August 1995 with the goal of establishing an innovative treatment approach that would emphasize the value delivery of treatment and services and maximize future market "success" and profitability. The team identified market segments, conducted survey research, and performed in-context customer interviews as part of their planning for this treatment system. The target for completion of a fully operational clinic was the summer of 1996. This paper summarizes the process and results of the project to date through the spring of 1995 and offers conclusions about the value of the CIDM/QFD methodology for strategic planning of healthcare services.

Article 28. *Reposable Medical Device Development: Creatively Meeting Customers' Needs (Conjoint Analysis & QFD)* George J. Marcel, Heidi Youngkin, and Bob Anthony.

Healthcare Company: Guidant—Origin Medsystems, Inc. (USA)

Abstract: This case study provides the initial results on integrating marketing and quality tools in a medical device application—a resposable (partially reusable, partially disposable) instrument used in Minimum Invasive Surgery (MIS). It addresses how use of combined disciplines can provide an improved product and capture a sense of urgency. The urgency is to bring to market a product that meets or exceeds the customer requirements in whole—quality, cost, and timing. The integration tools included: Market analysis survey—conjoint analysis; Concurrent engineering—specification development/QFD; Design for use—product innovation; Design for manufacture; Total cost; and Regulatory compliance.

Article 30. *Quality Function Deployment and Product and Process Reliability,* Ian Ferguson, Ian Ferguson Associates.

Healthcare Institution/Company: Not Specified

Abstract: One of the major benefits of QFD beyond the first phase of the House of Quality is the identification of key characteristics and features that provide a customer base for the Engineering functional requirements. This vital information can then be tested both in the Concept Selection stage and in the Product and Process design stage for both performance and reliability. This paper concentrates on the Reliability program, showing how Test planning is achieved and the use of Risk analysis tools such as Fault Tree Analysis, and Failure Mode and Effects Analysis, both at the Concept Selection stage and also at the Product and Process Design stage.

The paper also shows how this information is used with Experimental Design, in both Product and Process design, to ensure robustness of design to uncontrollable events. The methods used in this paper are illustrated by case studies from the Automotive, Healthcare, and Software Engineering Industries.

Number 9/1997

Article 5. *Prioritizing Customer Requirements in a Rapidly Changing Market Using Market Driven Product Definition,* William F. Naccarato

Healthcare Company: Dade International, Inc.

Abstract: Dade International, Inc., applied a QFD based systematic process "Market Driven Product Definition" for the identification and prioritization of customer requirements, assessment of the competition relative to those requirements, and the development of metrics to assess when those requirements have been met to the development of an analyzer for hospital clinical laboratories. The article reviews changes in the healthcare market due to significant pressures to reduce cost that are affecting the clinical laboratory. The paper focuses on the prioritization step methods of the process, and describes the results of surveys and Kano questionnaires to quantify customer-satisfaction levels related to specific requirements.

Article 9. *A QFD-Based Evaluation of Prevention Services,* Robert F. Hales, ProAction Development, Inc.; Pamela Clark and Don Lakes of TriHealth Systems.

Healthcare Institution: TriHealth (partnership between Bethesda Hospitals and Good Samaritan Hospital, Cincinnati, Ohio)

Abstract: In a changing healthcare environment, payors and providers of services including healthcare organizations, physicians, and employers are refocusing their efforts on health services that are designed to prevent or minimize the impact of illness or injury. This paper describes the QFD-derived process used by a cross-functional team at TriHealth charged with the task of developing recommendations on an overall corporate strategy and structure for the delivery of preventive services. Their research, analysis, and development of recommendations were driven by the program, service, configuration, and organization Measures identified to assure delivery of prioritized benefits for all of TriHealth's customer sets.

Number 10/1998

Article 3: *A Case Study Using Quality Function Deployment and Failure Mode and Effects Analysis in the Design of a Drug Delivery Device,* Phil Price, Novartis Pharma AG, Ian Ferguson, Ian Ferguson Associates.

Healthcare Company: Novartis Pharma AG

Abstract: This paper describes a robust design process integrating QFD, the Business Model/Plan, Concept Selection and Failure and Risk Analysis methods such as FMEA into the design and development of medical products and manufacturing processes. Specific methods to integrate these design techniques with Functional Analysis, concept development, prototyping and design evaluation are described and related to recent European Medical Device Directives.

Article 18. *Innovation and Customer Focus: A Medical Marketing Success Study Demonstrating TRIZ and QFD,* Ellen Domb, The PQR Group, David Corbin, Delcor Interactives International, Inc.

Healthcare Company: Delcor Interactives International, Inc.

Abstract: This case study illustrates the iterative combination of QFD, TRIZ, medical business experience, and entrepreneurial intuition that have gone into a successful new business venture. Through use of the technical tools of product development with the founders' intuition and experience, the development and marketing of a unique family of medical products and services have rapidly gone from concept, to prototype, to test market, to nationwide distribution and sales.

Article 23. *An Application of Quality Function in the Medical Device Industry,* Dr. Shihab Asfour, Dr. Eleftherios Iakovou, the Department of Industrial Engineering, University of Miami. Gilbert Cortes, Dade Behring.

Healthcare Company: Dade Behring

Abstract: This article provides an overview of the medical device development environment and the potential utility of QFD in that arena. Medical Device Design Requirements and Critical Factors are discussed, with a review of the relations of FDA guidelines and ISO 9000 standards on design controls. The application of QFD to the development of an in vitro diagnostic analyzer is presented as a case study, with a focus on the importance of "mean time between failures" (MTBF) as an engineering attribute related to key customer-demanded qualities. The use of robust design to successfully extend MTBF is detailed.

Article 30. *A Hospital-Based Service Example of QFD,* Edward Chaplin, M. D.

Healthcare Institution: Continentinal Rehabilitation Hospital of San Diego

Abstract: The article reviews a project to incorporate a customer focus into a rehabilitation hospital service that provides multidisciplinary evaluations of complex and/or catastrophic injuries. The service is low in volume, complex, provider intensive, and involves multiple business entities (suppliers). The project included the following: (1) Classic Quality Function Deployment–Customer Deployment, capturing the Voice of the Customer, Quality Deployment, Functional Deployment, Reliability Deployment,

New Process, and Task Deployment; (2) an example of using reinforcing (positive) feedback to self-organize and self-regulate the management of provider commitments, which, in turn, enhanced the effectiveness, reliability, and robustness of a deployed process; (3) an example where the use of the concepts from ARIZ broke through apparent incompatibilities between demanded qualities of the injured person and the insurance regulations.

Number 11/1999

Article 18: *Using TRIZ as a Creative Process for Breaking Mindpatterns,* Tore Wiik.

Healthcare Company: Fraunhufer Technology Development Group

Abstract: Two successful cases in which TRIZ has been used extensively are discussed. TRIZ has first been used as a tool to stimulate group creativity so that a large number of alternatives have been generated. Then the methodology has been used as a tool to find actual solutions using the classical TRIZ tools for sterilizing equipment for drugs and next generation cutting tool holders.

Other References
Mazur, G. 1993. "Quality Function Deployment for a Medical Device." IEEE Symposium on Computer-Based Medical Systems, 10–15.

Abstract: A report on the use of QFD in the development of an endotracheal tube for use in laser otolaryngologic surgery. Customer needs and demanded qualities were identified; quality characteristics were evaluated and used to rate competitive products. Key design characteristics and concepts led to successful development and market introduction.

Radharamanan, R. 1996. "Quality Function Deployment as Applied to a Healthcare System." *Computers and Ind. Eng.* (UK) 31, 1–2, (October) 443–64. We used QFD to help plan Karuna Hospice here in Brisbane. Karuna is a palliative care organization that helps dying patients who wish to stay at home rather than go to the hospital. Karuna provides nursing and volunteer assistance to patients and their families. The organization was quite small, but we undertook detailed qualitative and quantitative market research on external and internal customer requirements.

Walker M.N. 1995. "Quality Function Deployment at Karuna Hospice Service." *Quality Australia* (July\August).

References

Action Workflow. Alameda, Calif. 94501: Action Technologies, Inc.

Akao, Y. 1989. *Quality Function Deployment: Integrating Customer Requirements into Product Design*. Portland, Ore.: Productivity Press.

Belasco, J. 1990. *Teaching the Elephant to Dance: Empowering Change in Your Organization*. New York: Crown Publishers, Inc.

Business Design Associates. 2200 Powell Street, Emeryville, Calif. 94608.

Chaplin, E. 1996. "Reengineering in Healthcare: Chain Handoff and the Four-Phase Work Cycle." *Quality Progress* 29(10):105–7.

——— et al. 1999. "Using Quality Function Deployment to Capture the Voice of the Customer and Translate It into the Voice of the Provider." *Journal of Joint Commission on Quality Improvement* 300–315.

——— et al. 1997. "The Importance of Negative Feedback and Consequences for Actions in the Design of Processes." *Quality Management in Healthcare* 6:70–74.

De Groot, A. 1946. *Thought and Choice in Chess*. New York: Mouton.

Dell, M., and C. Fredman. 1999. *Direct from Dell: Strategies That Revolutionized an Industry*. San Francisco: Harper Business.

Dunham, R. 1991. "Business Design Technology, Software Development for Customer Satisfaction." Proceedings of the twenty-fourth Annual Hawaii International Conference on System Sciences, Vol. III: 792.

Einhorn, E. 1992. "Expert Measurement and Mechanical Combination." *Organizational Behavior and Human Performance* 7:86, 106.

Fields, H. C. 1987. *Pain*. New York: McGraw-Hill.

FMEA: Potential Failure Mode and Effects Analysis. 2d Ed. 1995. Chrysler Corporation, Ford Motors Company, General Motors Corporation, Automotive Industry Action Group.

Fritz, R. 1996. *Corporate Tides: The Inescapable Laws of Organizational Structure*. San Francisco: Berrett-Koehler.

Gazzaniga, M.S. 1978. *The Integrated Mind*. New York: Plenum Press.

———. 1980. *The Bisected Brain*. New York: Appleton-Century Crofts.

Granger, C. V., et al. 1990. "Functional Assessment Scales: A Study of Persons with Multiple Sclerosis." *Archives of Physical Medicine Rehabilitation* 71:870–75.

Gregory, R.L. 1966. *Eye and Brain: The Psychology of Seeing*. New York: McGraw-Hill.

Institute of Medicine. 1985. *Assessing Medical Technologies*. Washington, D.C.: National Academy Press, Office of Technology Assessment.

Johnson, M. 1993. *Moral Imagination, Implications of Cognitive Science for Ethics*. Chicago: The University of Chicago Press.

Kahaneman, D., and A. Tversky. 1982. "On the Statistical Intuitions." *Cognition* 11:123–41.

Kano's Method. 1993. "A Special Edition on Kano's Methods for Understanding Customer-Defined Quality." *The Center for Quality Management Journal* 2(4) (Fall). 2–36.

Kaplan, S. 1996. *An Introduction to TRIZ: The Russian Theory of Inventive Problem Solving*. Southfield, Mich.: Ideation International, Inc.

Kauffman, D. 1980. *Systems One: An Introduction to Systems Thinking*. Cambridge, Mass.: Future Systems, Inc.

Kauffman, S. 1993. *The Origins of Order*. New York: Oxford University Press.

King, B. 1989. *Better Designs in Half the Time: Implementing Quality Function Deployment in America*. Methuen, Mass.: Goal/QPC.

Klein, G. 1999. *Sources of Power: How People Make Decisions*. Cambridge: The MIT Press.

Kübler-Ross, E. 1997 (Reprint Ed.). *On Death and Dying*. New York: Collier Books.

Levine, J. D., N. C. Gordon, T. R. Jones, and H. C. Fields. 1978. "The Narcotic Antagonist Naloxone Enhances Clinical Pain." *Nature* 272:826.

Lipet, B. 1993. *Neurophysiology of Consciousness-Selected Papers and New Essays by Benjamin Lipet*. Boston, Mass.: Birkhauser.

Lippitt, G. L. 1982. "Managing Conflict in Today's Organizations." *Training and Development Journal* (July): 67–74.

Manturana, H. R., and F. J. Varela. 1988. *The Tree of Knowledge*. Boston: Shambhala, New Science Library.

Mazur, G. H. 1996. *Comprehensive Quality Function Deployment Service Version V 5.0*. Ann Arbor, Mich.: Japan Business Consultants *(gmazur@engin.umich.edu)*.

Meehl, P. 1965(1955). "Seer Over Sign: The First Good Example." *Journal of Experimental Research in Personality* 1:27–32.

Nakui, S. 1991. "Comprehensive QFD." The transactions of the Third Symposium on QFD, Novi, Mich.

Nayatani, Y., et al. 1988. *The Seven New Quality Tools: Practical Applications for Managers*. Translated by John Loftus. Toyko: Juse Press.

Ohno, T. 1988. *Toyota Production System: Beyond Large-Scale Production*. Portland, Ore.: Productivity Press.

Palmer, B. 1999. "Click Here for Decisions." *Fortune* 139:153–56.

Pribram, K. 1991. *Brain and Perception*. Hillsdale, N.J.: Lawrence Erlbaum Associates.

Pugh, S. 1991. *Total Design: Integrated Methods for Successful Product Engineering*. Reading, Mass. Addison-Wesley.

Ramachandran, V. S. 1993. "Filling in Gaps in Perception: Part 2. Scotomas and Phantom Limbs." *Current Directions in Psychology* 2:56, 65.

Saaty, T. L. 1993. *Decision Making for Leaders: The Analytical Hierarchy Process of Decisions in a Complex World*. Pittsburgh, Penn.: RWS Publications.

Spinosa, C, Flores, F and Dreyfus, H, Disclosing New Worlds, MIT Press, Boston 1997.

Terninko, J. 1989. *Robust Design: Key Points for World-Class Quality.* Nottingham, N.H.: Responsible Management.

———. 1995. *Step-by-Step QFD: Customer-Driven Product Design.* Boca Raton, Fla.: St. Lucie Press.

——— et al. 1998. *Systematic Innovation: An Introduction to TRIZ.* Boca Raton, Fla.: St. Lucie Press.

Zultner, R. E. 1992. "Quality Function Deployment (QFD) for Software: Satisfying Customers." *American Programmer* (February). 12–22.

———. 1993. "Blitz QFD" in Tutorials Tenth Quality Function Deployment Synposium. Novi, MI.

Index